T0263141

Hematology

Editors

MARY LOU WARREN
MELISSA MCLENON

CRITICAL CARE NURSING CLINICS OF NORTH AMERICA

www.ccnursing.theclinics.com

Consulting Editor
JAN FOSTER

December 2013 • Volume 25 • Number 4

ELSEVIER

1600 John F. Kennedy Boulevard • Suite 1800 • Philadelphia, Pennsylvania, 19103-2899

http://www.theclinics.com

CRITICAL CARE NURSING CLINICS OF NORTH AMERICA Volume 25, Number 4
December 2013 ISSN 0899-5885, ISBN-13: 978-0-323-28654-1

Editor: Kerry Holland
Developmental Editor: Stephanie Carter

© 2013 Elsevier Inc. All rights reserved.

This periodical and the individual contributions contained in it are protected under copyright by Elsevier, and the following terms and conditions apply to their use:

Photocopying
Single photocopies of single articles may be made for personal use as allowed by national copyright laws. Permission of the Publisher and payment of a fee is required for all other photocopying, including multiple or systematic copying, copying for advertising or promotional purposes, resale, and all forms of document delivery. Special rates are available for educational institutions that wish to make photocopies for non-profit educational classroom use. For information on how to seek permission visit www.elsevier.com/permissions or call: (+44) 1865 843830 (UK)/(+1) 215 239 3804 (USA).

Derivative Works
Subscribers may reproduce tables of contents or prepare lists of articles including abstracts for internal circulation within their institutions. Permission of the Publisher is required for resale or distribution outside the institution. Permission of the Publisher is required for all other derivative works, including compilations and translations (please consult www.elsevier.com/permissions).

Electronic Storage or Usage
Permission of the Publisher is required to store or use electronically any material contained in this periodical, including any article or part of an article (please consult www.elsevier.com/permissions). Except as outlined above, no part of this publication may be reproduced, stored in a retrieval system or transmitted in any form or by any means, electronic, mechanical, photocopying, recording or otherwise, without prior written permission of the Publisher.

Notice
No responsibility is assumed by the Publisher for any injury and/or damage to persons or property as a matter of products liability, negligence or otherwise, or from any use or operation of any methods, products, instructions or ideas contained in the material herein. Because of rapid advances in the medical sciences, in particular, independent verification of diagnoses and drug dosages should be made.

Although all advertising material is expected to conform to ethical (medical) standards, inclusion in this publication does not constitute a guarantee or endorsement of the quality or value of such product or of the claims made of it by its manufacturer.

Critical Care Nursing Clinics of North America (ISSN 0899-5885) is published quarterly by Elsevier Inc., 360 Park Avenue South, New York, NY 10010-1710. Months of issue are March, June, September, and December. Business and Editorial Offices: 1600 John F. Kennedy Blvd., Suite 1800, Philadelphia, PA 19103-2899. Periodicals postage paid at New York, NY and additional mailing offices. Subscription prices are $150.00 per year for US individuals, $328.00 per year for US institutions, $80.00 per year for US students and residents, $200.00 per year for Canadian individuals, $412.00 per year for Canadian institutions, $230.00 per year for international individuals, $412.00 per year for international institutions and $115.00 per year for Canadian and international students/residents. To receive student/resident rate, orders must be accompanied by name of affiliated institution, data of term, and the signature of program/residency coordinator on institution letterhead. Orders will be billed at individual rate until proof of status is received. Foreign air speed delivery is included in all Clinics subscription prices. All prices are subject to change without notice. **POSTMASTER:** Send address changes to Critical Care Nursing Clinics of North America, Elsevier Health Sciences Division, Subscription Customer Service, 3251 Riverport Lane, Maryland Heights, MO 63043. **Customer Service: 1-800-654-2452 (US and Canada); 314-447-8871 (outside US and Canada). Fax: 314-447-8029. E-mail: JournalsCustomerService-usa@elsevier.com (for print support) and JournalsOnlineSupport-usa@elsevier.com (for online support).**

Reprints. For copies of 100 or more of articles in this publication, please contact the Commercial Reprints Department, Elsevier Inc., 360 Park Avenue South, New York, New York, 10010-1710; Tel.: 212-633-3874, Fax: 212-633-3820, and E-mail: reprints@elsevier.com.

Critical Care Nursing Clinics of North America is covered in MEDLINE/PubMed (Index Medicus), International Nursing Index, Nursing Citation Index, Cumulative Index to Nursing and Allied Health Literature, and RNdex Top 100.

Printed and bound by CPI Group (UK) Ltd, Croydon, CR0 4YY

Transferred to digital print 2012

Contributors

CONSULTING EDITOR

JAN FOSTER, PhD, RN, CNS
College of Nursing, Texas Woman's University, Houston, Texas

EDITORS

MARY LOU WARREN, DNP, RN, CNS-CC
Advanced Practice Nurse, Department of Critical Care, M.D. Anderson Cancer Center, Houston, Texas

MELISSA MCLENON, DNP, APRN, ACNP
Advanced Practice Nurse, University of Maryland Medical Center, Cardiac Surgery Critical Care, Baltimore, Maryland

AUTHORS

JACQUELINE B. BROADWAY-DUREN, MSN, FNP-C
Family Nurse Practitioner, Department of Leukemia, University of Texas MD Anderson Cancer Center, Houston, Texas

EDYTHE M. (LYN) GREENBERG, PhD, RN, FNP-BC
Department of Leukemia, MD Anderson Cancer Center, Houston, Texas

ROBERT HANKS, PhD, FNP-C, RNC
Assistant Professor-Clinical, Academic Project Manager, Graduate Nurse Education Demonstration Project, School of Nursing, University of Texas Health Science Center at Houston, Houston, Texas

JENNIFER K. JOHNSON, MSN, RN, ACNS-BC, AOCNS
Nocturnal Mid-Level Provider, Nocturnal Program, MD Anderson Cancer Center, The University of Texas, Houston, Texas

ELIZABETH S. (SUE) KALED, MS, RN, NP-C, FNP-BC
Department of Leukemia, MD Anderson Cancer Center, Houston, Texas

HILLARY KLAASSEN, PA-C
Physician Assistant, Department of Leukemia, University of Texas MD Anderson Cancer Center, Houston, Texas

CAROLE L. MACKAVEY, RN, MSN, FNP-C
Doctoral Student, University of Texas Health Science Center at Houston, Houston, Texas

JULIA A. MANNING, MSN, RN, CCRN, ACNP-BC
Director of Clinical Operations, Woodlands North Houston Heart Center, Houston, Texas

ALEXANDRA PROBST, MS, PA-C
Department of Leukemia, MD Anderson Cancer Center, Houston, Texas

ELIZABETH SORENSEN, MSN, RN, ACNS-BC, AOCNS
Advanced Practice Nurse, Lymphoma and Myeloma Department, MD Anderson Cancer Center, The University of Texas, Houston, Texas

KATY M. TOALE, PharmD, BCPS
Clinical Pharmacy Specialist, Department of Pharmacy, MD Anderson Cancer Center, Houston, Texas

Contents

Anemias continue to present a challenge to the health care profession. Anemia is defined as a reduction in one or more of the RBC indices. Patients presenting with a mild form of anemia may be asymptomatic; however, in more serious cases the anemia can become life threatening. In many cases the clinical presentation also reflects the underlying cause. Anemia may be attributed to various causes, whereas autoimmune RBC destruction may be attributed to intrinsic and extrinsic factors. Laboratory tests are essential in facilitating early detection and differentiation of anemia.

Thrombocytopenia is defined as a platelet count less than 150,000/μL. It can be the result of decreased platelet production, sequestration of the platelets, or increased destruction of the platelets. The clinical presentation may vary from an incidental finding to obvious bleeding. Causes of thrombocytopenia include infections, malignancy, liver disease, autoimmune disorders, disseminated intravascular coagulation, pregnancy, medications, and coagulation disorders. Treatment is determined by the underlying cause of the thrombocytopenia. This article discusses the evaluation and management of common causes of thrombocytopenia.

Coagulopathy-related bleeding events are a major concern in the management of acute and chronic liver disease. The liver attempts to maintain a balance between procoagulant and anticoagulant factors, and providers struggle with poor prognostic indicators to manage bleeding and critical complications. Subtle changes in patient presentation that may require extensive provider-directed interventions, such as blood transfusions, intravenous fluid management, mitigating possible sepsis, and evaluating appropriate pharmacologic treatment, are discussed.

Lymphoma presents itself from slow growing and asymptomatic to aggressive and destructive. Suspicion of aggressive lymphoma warrants prompt diagnostic evaluation because the tumor can be extremely fast growing and can cause significant sequelae including but not limited to tissue damage, immune suppression, organ failure, compromised circulation, and death. The standard evaluation includes laboratory assay, infectious disease panel, radiographic imaging with computed tomography, bone marrow biopsy, and tissue diagnosis. Two cases studies are presented describing the range of different acute issues that may arise with aggressive lymphomas including tumor lysis, HIV, small bowel obstruction, superior vena cava compression, aggressive disease transformation, and acute renal injury.

CRITICAL CARE NURSING CLINICS OF NORTH AMERICA

DOWNLOAD
Free App!

Review Articles
THE CLINICS

NOW AVAILABLE FOR YOUR iPhone and iPad

Preface

Hematologic Issues in Critically Ill Patients

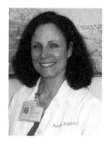 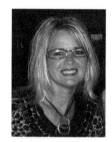

Mary Lou Warren, DNP, RN, CNS-CC   Melissa McLenon, DNP, APRN, ACNP
Editors

Clinicians are often challenged by the complexity of hematologic issues affecting critically and acutely ill patients. As research in this field continues to thrive, the understanding and management of these hematologic anomalies allow the clinician to be more astute in the recognition and treatment of these conditions. A variety of patient populations are more prone to developing hematologic issues, including those with cardiac, liver, infectious, and oncologic diseases. This issue of *Critical Care Nursing Clinics of North America* addresses some of the more common hematologic issues that critically ill patients face. The authors discuss the recognition, diagnosis, management, and challenges of a variety of conditions affecting this patient population. As clinicians, we must be prepared to thoroughly evaluate and treat hematologic conditions, such as anemias, thrombocytopenias, and coagulopathies. Our goal is to provide a foundation of knowledge in which the clinician can apply in daily practice in order to provide the highest quality of care for this specialized patient population.

Mary Lou Warren, DNP, RN, CNS-CC
Advanced Practice Nurse
Department of Critical Care
M.D. Anderson Cancer Center, 1515 Holcombe Boluevard
Houston, TX 21030, USA

Melissa McLenon, DNP, APRN, ACNP
Advanced Practice Nurse
University of Maryland Medical Center
Cardiac Surgery Critical Care, 22 S. Greene Street
Baltimore, MD 21201, USA

E-mail addresses:
mlwarren@mdanderson.org (M.L. Warren)
mmclenon@umm.edu (M. McLenon)

Crit Care Nurs Clin N Am 25 (2013) ix
http://dx.doi.org/10.1016/j.ccell.2013.09.010
0899-5885/13/$ – see front matter © 2013 Elsevier Inc. All rights reserved.
ccnursing.theclinics.com

Anemias

Jacqueline B. Broadway-Duren, MSN, FNP-C*, Hillary Klaassen, PA-C

KEYWORDS

- Anemia • Hemoglobin • Hematocrit • Autoimmune hemolytic anemia (AIHA)
- Sickle cell anemia (SCA) • Sickle cell disease (SCD) • Iron deficiency • B_{12} deficiency

KEY POINTS

- Anemias present significant expense and challenges to the US health care system.
- The focus of future research is primarily genetic research and associated risk factors that predispose patients to anemias.
- It is imperative that health care providers are made aware of various types of anemia and the appropriate management options.
- Research is ongoing regarding various aspects of anemia.

INTRODUCTION

The healthcare industry in the United States (US) is faced with many complex illnesses. Among those complex illnesses exist a variety of anemias. Anemia is a condition characterized by a decreased number of circulating red blood cells (RBCs) and/or hemoglobin. This article discusses various types of anemia, clinical characteristics, and evidence-based management strategies.

Erythrocytes (RBCs) facilitate circulation of oxygen from the lungs to vital organs. The average, healthy adult needs a large number of RBCs to fulfill this role, approximately 5 million RBCs per microliter of blood. Anemia can be defined as either a reduced number of circulating RBCs, reduced hemoglobin concentration, or reduced hematocrit (HCT).[1] Anemia is commonly found worldwide, resulting from numerous causes.

This article provides an overview of RBC production, definitions of anemia, clinical presentation, appropriate diagnostic laboratory evaluation, and methods utilized to determine causes of anemia. Anemia is a complex subject matter, however, the article focuses on 4 common types of anemia: (1) iron-deficient anemia, (2) vitamin B_{12}–deficient anemia, (3) sickle cell anemia (SCA), and (4) hemolytic anemia.

Financial Disclosure: Jacqueline Broadway-Duren and Hillary Klaassen have no financial disclosures to report.
Department of Leukemia, University of Texas MD Anderson Cancer Center, 1515 Holcombe Boulevard, Houston, TX 77030, USA
* Corresponding author.
E-mail address: jbbroadw@mdanderson.org

RBC PRODUCTION

The production of RBCs in the bone marrow (BM) is stimulated by a hormone released from the kidneys called erythropoietin (EPO). While in the BM, RBCs must grow and differentiate from erythroid progenitors into reticulocytes and eventually into mature RBCs. Contained within each RBC is a protein that is able to link to oxygen and then release it in tissue capillaries. RBCs circulate in the blood for approximately 120 days and are then removed from circulation by macrophages.[1]

In order to maintain a balance between production and loss of RBCs, in a steady state the BM must produce 50,000 reticulocytes/μL of whole blood each day.[1] However, in the event of an increased loss of blood (eg, acute hemorrhage, gastrointestinal [GI] bleed, or hemolytic anemia), and the bone marrow does not effectively compensate with increased RBC production to meet the demands, the patient will inevitably develop anemia.

CATEGORIZING ANEMIA

The explanations for anemia are numerous; therefore, a methodological approach for determining the cause of anemia should be considered by clinicians, especially in complicated cases of anemia. Two approaches are utilized in determining the causality of anemia: the kinetic approach and the morphologic approach.

KINETIC APPROACH

The kinetic approach examines the causative mechanism that produces the decrease in hemoglobin and is divided into 3 categories: (1) increased loss of RBCs, (2) increased destruction of RBCs, and (3) decreased production of RBCs.[2]

Increased loss of RBCs may result from a chronic or acute hemorrhage. Blood loss can be obvious in cases like traumatic injuries, heavy menstruation, hematemesis, gross hematuria, or melena stools. However, occult blood loss is less obvious in cases such as slow-bleeding ulcers or GI cancers and can only be detected with further diagnostic testing.

Causes of increased destruction of RBCs include; hemolytic anemias that are either inherited (eg, sickle cell disease [SCD], thalassemia) or acquired (eg, autoimmune hemolytic anemia, malaria, splenomegaly, hemolytic uremic syndrome) (**Table 1**).

Decreased production of RBCs can be caused by lack of essential vitamins or hormones needed for normal erythropoiesis or by bone marrow disease. Iron, vitamin B_{12}, and folic acid deficiencies are classic examples of nutrient deficiencies that cause anemia. Hormones are also important in regulating hematopoiesis. Patients with chronic renal failure can develop anemia if the kidneys do not produce the erythropoietin levels that are needed to increase erythropoiesis (see **Table 1**). Other hormone deficiencies, such as hypothyroidism and hypogonadism, can also lead to anemia.[3] Decreased RBC production may also result from bone marrow suppression from chemotherapy, radiation therapy, or from disease within the bone marrow (eg, myelodysplastic syndrome, aplastic anemia, tumor infiltration).[4]

MORPHOLOGIC APPROACH

The morphologic approach categorizes anemia by RBC size using the mean corpuscular volume (MCV). The morphologic approach has 3 categories: (1) microcytic anemia, in which the MCV is less than 80 fL; (2) normocytic anemia, in which the MCV is within the normal range of 80 to 100 fL; and (3) macrocytic anemia, in which the MCV is greater than 100 fL (**Table 2**).[5]

Table 1
Kinetic approach to anemia

Investigating Anemia

Decreased RBC production	Decreased nutrients • Iron, vitamin B$_{12}$, or folate deficiency Bone marrow disorders • Aplastic anemia • Tumor infiltration • Myelodysplastic syndrome Bone marrow suppression • Drug effects • Chemotherapy and/or radiation Decreased hormones • Erythropoietin • Hypothyroidism • Hypogonadism
Increased RBC destruction	Inherited hemolytic anemias • Hereditary spherocytosis • G6PD deficiency • Hemoglobinopathies (eg, SCD, thalassemias) Acquired hemolytic anemias • Autoimmune hemolytic anemia • Infections (eg, malaria, *Babesia*, *Bartonella*) • Live disease • Hypersplenism • Microangiopathy (eg, hemolytic uremic syndrome) • Transfusion reactions (eg, ABO incompatibility)
Increase RBC loss	• Trauma • GI bleed • Slow bleeding ulcer or carcinoma • Menorrhagia

Abbreviation: G6PD, glucose-6-phosphte dehydrogenase.

Table 2
Morphologic approach to anemia

Investigating Anemia	Causes
Microcytic (MCV<80 fL)	Iron deficiency Copper deficiency Thalassemias Hemoglobinopathies Anemia of chronic disease (inflammation)
Normocytic (MCV 80–100 fL)	Acute blood loss Anemia of chronic disease Chronic renal failure Hypothyroidism Bone marrow suppression (eg, RBC aplasia, aplastic anemia)
Macrocytic (MCV>100 fL)	Vitamin B$_{12}$ (cobalamin) deficiency Folate deficiency Alcohol abuse Myelodysplastic syndrome Aplastic anemia Reticulocytosis (eg, in response to hemolysis, blood loss) Drug-induced anemia (eg, hydroxyurea, methotrexate, 6-mercaptopurine)

Microcytic anemia is characterized by small RBCs containing decreased hemoglobin content, making them hypochromic. The most common types of microcytic anemias include iron-deficient anemia, α-thalassemia or β-thalassemia minor, and anemia of chronic disease. Macrocytic anemias are characterized by large RBCs, resultant from abnormal nucleic acid metabolism or RBC maturation.[6] Examples of macrocytic anemias are listed in **Table 2**.

CLINICAL PRESENTATION

The most common symptom of anemia is fatigue. Other symptoms can include dyspnea with exertion or at rest, weakness, palpitations, and hearing roaring in the ears. More serious complications can develop, such as angina, arrhythmias, congestive heart failure, and even myocardial infarction in some cases.[7] The severity of symptoms depends on oxygen demands, rate of onset, and degree of anemia. For example, those who develop anemia over an extended period of time may not be as cognizant of symptoms; however, significant improvement in health and well-being occurs with the onset of treatment.

Physical examination can also play an essential role in diagnosing anemia. Clinical findings, such as; pallor of the skin, conjunctivae, lips, palmar creases, and nail beds, should increase suspicion of anemia and warrant laboratory testing.[8] Other key physical findings on investigation of anemia, include: postural hypotension secondary to intravascular volume loss, jaundice caused by hemolytic anemia, and bone pain and/or organomegaly with infiltrative disease of the bone marrow.[1]

Obtaining a detailed history is crucial when investigating the cause of anemia. In premenopausal patients, frequency and duration of menses are key elements to explore. In postmenopausal or male patients, ascertaining a history of abdominal pain, reflux disease, peptic ulcer disease, or frequent use of nonsteroidal antiinflammatory drugs (NSAIDs) is significant. Furthermore, past history of bleeding (eg, hematochezia, melena stools, gross hematuria, hematemesis) should be noted. The clinician should also inquire whether any history of autoimmune conditions, malignancies, or family history of thalassemia or SCD exists.

DIAGNOSIS

Anemia can be defined as either a reduced number of circulating RBCs, reduced hemoglobin concentration, or reduced HCT. Hemoglobin is the oxygen-carrying pigment in each erythrocyte and hemoglobin concentration is a measurement of the concentration of hemoglobin to whole blood. HCT is a percentage of RBCs occupying whole blood. The World Health Organization (WHO) defines anemia as a hemoglobin B less than 13 g/dL or an HCT less than 41% in men and an hemoglobin B less than 12 g/dL or an HCT less than 36% in women.[9]

Initial laboratory evaluation of an anemia includes complete blood count and differential, which routinely includes RBC count, RBC indices, hemoglobin B, HCT, platelets, white blood cell (WBC) count with differential, reticulocyte count, and peripheral blood smear. Depending on these results, additional diagnostic labs may be added (eg, bone marrow biopsy in the presence of pancytopenia, iron studies in the presence of microcytic anemia).[9]

IRON DEFICIENCY ANEMIA

Iron is an element needed for hemoglobin synthesis and is essential in contributing to oxygen-carrying ability to RBCs. A lack of proper iron stores eventually leads to inadequate hemoglobin and erythrocyte production, thus resulting in microcytic anemia.

Iron deficiency anemia (IDA) is the predominant form of anemia worldwide.[10] In the United States, 5% of women and 2% of men have iron-deficient anemia.[11,12] Iron deficiency is the result of inadequate iron consumption, decreased iron absorption from the gut, or iron loss secondary to gross or occult blood loss. Replacing iron stores and correcting anemia with iron supplementation is easy and effective. However, it is crucial to investigate the cause of iron deficiency because, in some cases, it can be life threatening (eg, colon cancer) and may require prompt treatment.

IRON METABOLISM AND STORAGE

The adult human body contains a total of 3 to 4 g of iron.[10] The body is able to tightly regulate iron storage because iron overload can be toxic, whereas iron deficiency leads to anemia. In general, the daily amount of iron absorbed should equal the daily amount of iron lost.[13] Humans consume 2 different forms of iron: (1) heme iron, which is found in meat and is easily absorbed; and (2) nonheme iron, found in cereals, vegetables, and beans and not as easily absorbed. Once absorbed into the blood stream, iron is transported by transferrin to the bone marrow for hemoglobin synthesis and production of RBCs.[10] RBCs circulate for approximately 120 days before being phagocytized by macrophages and the remaining heme iron is then recycled to make new RBCs. Recycled iron from degraded erythrocytes is the primary source of iron for erythropoiesis.[14]

Iron exists in multiple forms in the human body: in the hemoglobin molecule, bound to and transported by transferrin, and stored as ferritin. High quantities of iron are stored in the liver, spleen, and bone marrow for future erythropoiesis.[15] However, when more iron is lost than absorbed by the body, these iron stores become depleted over time and the person becomes iron deficient. IDA occurs when the deficit is severe enough to negatively affect erythropoiesis.

CLINICAL PRESENTATION

The clinical picture of IDA depends on the severity of iron deficiency and the rate of the onset of anemia. The most common symptoms of generalized anemia include fatigue, weakness, exercise intolerance, shortness of breath, and poor concentration. There are some iron-deficient patients who also experience alopecia, spoon nails (koilonychias), atrophic glossitis, or restless leg syndrome.[16,17] Severely iron-deficient patients can also develop pica, an almost irresistible urge to eat nonnutritive substances such as ice, clay, or paper. Pica for ice is considered specific for iron deficiency and patients with this eating disorder should be evaluated for IDA immediately.[18,19]

DIAGNOSIS

The gold standard for diagnosing IDA is a bone marrow biopsy to assess iron stores.[20] However, because this method is costly and invasive, most outpatient physicians instead rely on clinical findings and peripheral blood work to make the diagnosis. Classic laboratory findings in patients with IDA include microcytic anemia, hypochromic erythrocytes, low serum iron levels, low serum ferritin, low percent saturation of transferrin, and high transferrin and total iron binding capacity (TIBC).[10] Among the aforementioned laboratory tests, the serum ferritin level (stored form of iron) is the most sensitive and specific blood test for assessing iron stores, in otherwise healthy adults is the serum ferritin level (storage form of iron).[21] A low serum ferritin level in the setting of anemia is usually diagnostic for iron deficiency anemia. When diagnosing IDA, tests should include complete blood count (CBC), RBC indices, serum iron levels, serum ferritin levels, percent saturation of transferrin, transferrin levels, and TIBC.

Once the diagnosis of IDA has been made it is necessary to investigate the cause (**Table 3**). Obtaining the patient history is important and can help guide further diagnostic testing. The most likely cause of iron-deficient anemia also depends on age and sex. In premenopausal women, excessive menstrual loss is the most likely cause. In pregnant women, there is an increased demand for iron supplementation that is likely not being met. In men and postmenopausal women, chronic GI bleeds are the most frequent cause of iron-deficient anemia.[13] The most concerning source of a GI bleed is from a cancerous lesion, such as colon cancer, and should be investigated immediately. For patients with a suspected GI bleed, a fecal occult blood test, colonoscopy, and upper endoscopy should be considered. Other tests to further investigate the cause of iron-deficient anemia may include a urinalysis to rule out hematuria or celiac blood test to rule out celiac sprue.

TREATMENT

The principal way to replenish iron stores after being diagnosed with IDA is to begin taking oral iron supplements. Increasing the consumption of meat and other iron rich foods may not be sufficient, depending on the severity of iron deficiency. The US Centers for Disease Control and Prevention (CDC) recommend 150 to 200 mg/d of elemental iron, to be taken in 2 to 3 divided doses a day.[22] Factors that optimize iron absorption include the acidic environment of the stomach and vitamin C.[10] Both increase the bioavailability of dietary iron so it is recommend to take iron supplements on an empty stomach or with a glass of orange juice. The benefit of oral therapy is that it is cost-effective. The hemoglobin usually improves within just 1 to 2 weeks of iron supplementation.[23] However, those who take oral iron supplements can experience abdominal discomfort, nausea, vomiting, and constipation. These common side effects can decrease patient compliance for those who need daily supplementation. In some patients, intravenous iron therapy can be considered if the patient is refractory to oral supplementation or intolerant.

Table 3 Causes of IDA	
Cause	**Causes**
Deficient intake	Malnourishment
	Increased demands for iron: pregnancy, lactation, adolescence
Decreased absorption	Celiac disease
	Gastrectomy
	Gastric bypass surgery
	Whipple disease
Increased loss	Frequent NSAID or aspirin use
	Peptic ulcer disease
	Helicobacter pylori gastritis
	GI cancers: esophagus, gastric, small bowel, or colorectal
	Inflammatory bowel disease: Crohn disease, ulcerative colitis
	Vascular lesions
	Excessive menstruation
	Intravascular hemolysis: prosthetic valves, marathon runners, Paroxysmal nocturnal hematuria

After initiating iron therapy, the next step is to address the underlying reason for the IDA (eg, cessation of regular NSAID use, treating *Helicobacter pylori* gastritis, surgery for colon cancer, gluten-free diet for those with celiac disease). These patients should be monitored over time to ensure that anemia has resolved and there has been adequate iron supplementation.

VITAMIN B$_{12}$ (COBALAMIN) DEFICIENCY

Vitamin B$_{12}$ (cobalamin) is an essential cofactor for nucleic acid and DNA production. It is not synthesized from plants and must be obtained mainly by consuming foods of animal origin. Cobalamin deficiency can develop if there is inadequate dietary intake (eg, strict vegans) or decreased absorption by the GI tract. The consequence is ineffective DNA production and development of megaloblastic anemia and neurodegenerative disease.[24]

Cobalamin deficiency is common worldwide and more prevalent among the elderly. It is estimated that 10% to 20% of the elderly are cobalamin deficient, mainly because of malabsorption, but only 5% to 10% are symptomatic.[25] A minimal threshold is required for diagnosing cobalamin deficiency, especially among the elderly and those with neurologic deficits.

CLINICAL PRESENTATION

Cobalamin-deficient patients have ineffective DNA synthesis, which can result in hematologic and neuropsychiatric deficits. These patients present with megaloblastic anemia (MCV>100 fL) and symptoms of anemia: fatigue, weakness, dyspnea, pallor appearance, tachycardia, and poor concentration. However, unique clinical findings associated with cobalamin deficiency can include glossitis and neurologic deficits on a physical examination. Glossitis is defined as a tongue that appears beefy red, swollen, and smooth, secondary to papillary atrophy. In addition, cobalamin-deficient patients may have bleeding gums. The second unique, and more serious, finding with severe cobalamin deficiency is neuropsychiatric deficits, which are caused by degeneration of the dorsal and lateral spinal columns and can lead to irreversible neurologic changes. Myelinopathy of these tracts can lead to paresthesia (numbness, tingling, or pain) of the extremities, loss of vibration and position sense, and hyperreflexia. Cerebellar changes can also lead to ataxia and cognitive deficits (eg, depression and dementia).[24] As cobalamin deficiency progresses it can also negatively affect hematopoiesis in all 3 cell lines in the bone marrow and eventually lead to pancytopenia.

CAUSES

Cobalamin deficiency is a result of either poor nutrition or poor absorption. Humans get most their cobalamin from consuming animal products. Therefore, those who are at high risk of developing cobalamin deficiency include vegetarians, vegans, or those who consume a minimal amount of meat, eggs, poultry, or dairy.

The second cause of cobalamin deficiency is poor absorption from the gut. Chronic alcoholism, Crohn disease, celiac disease, gastric bypass surgery, and long-term use of antacids all decrease the body's ability to absorb vitamin B$_{12}$. The most common cause for serious vitamin B$_{12}$ malabsorption is pernicious anemia, also known as autoimmune atrophic gastritis. Pernicious anemia is an autoimmune condition in which autoantibodies attack gastric parietal cells that produce intrinsic factor (intrinsic factor is a protein that binds to vitamin B$_{12}$ in the stomach and allows the body to absorb vitamin B$_{12}$ in the terminal ileum). Patients with pernicious anemia do not have intrinsic factor to bind to vitamin B_{12} for absorption and therefore have malabsorption and severe vitamin B_{12} deficiency. Patients with pernicious anemia need lifelong parenteral supplementation because they are unable to effectively absorb vitamin B_{12}.[26]

DIAGNOSIS

Patients with macrocytic (MCV>100 fL) anemia should be tested for potential vitamin B_{12} and folic acid deficiencies. Folic acid (vitamin B_9), like cobalamin (vitamin B_{12}), is essential for DNA synthesis, cellular growth, and regeneration. Cobalamin-deficient and folic acid–deficient patients both present with macrocytic anemia, therefore it is important to test for both types of vitamin deficiencies.

Diagnosis is based on the patient's history (eg, malabsorption, diet, family history of pernicious anemia or autoimmune conditions, symptoms) and physical examination (eg, neurologic deficits, hyperreflexia, glossitis, decreased vibration and position sense in lower extremities) in combination with laboratory findings. Blood tests should include a CBC with RBC indices, total serum cobalamin levels, homocysteine (Hcy), and methylmalonic acid (MMA) levels. A low threshold should exist in diagnosing cobalamin deficiency. Patients with macrocytic anemia and low or lower limit of normal total serum cobalamin levels likely have cobalamin deficiency.[26]

Hcy and MMA are both markedly increased in cobalamin-deficient patients. Between the two markers, MMA is more specific for detecting cobalamin deficiency, whereas Hcy can be increased in either the setting of folic acid or cobalamin-deficient states and is not specific.[27]

Even though increased MMA is specific for cobalamin deficiency, the diagnosis should not be based solely on increased MMA levels; MMA and Hcy are adjuvant tests that should be used to help confirm the already suspected diagnosis.

TREATMENT

Cobalamin deficiency that is caused by poor nutrition can be treated with high-dose oral Vitamin B_{12} replacement, 1000 to 2000 µg daily.[26] However, parenteral therapy is usually the preferred method of treatment, especially when the cause is poor absorption. It has also been argued that with parenteral therapy there is better compliance and monitoring. Those with severe vitamin B_{12} deficiencies should receive vitamin B_{12} intramuscular injections (1000 µg), with 8 to 10 loading doses, followed by monthly 1000-µg injections.[26]

Patients with pernicious anemia or significant malabsorption (eg, gastric bypass) should receive lifelong vitamin B_{12} supplementation. Adequate vitamin B_{12} replacement results in an almost immediate decrease in Hcy and MMA levels, within 2 months there is resolution of megaloblastic anemia, and within 6 months improvement/resolution of myelopathy.[26]

To summarize, most symptoms of vitamin B_{12} deficiency are reversible with timely, adequate supplementation. However, neurologic deficits may be permanent if not treated within 6 months of the onset of symptoms.[28] Only half of patients with neurologic changes respond to treatment, hence early recognition of cobalamin deficiency is critical.[25] There should be a low threshold for diagnosing vitamin B_{12} deficiency and beginning treatment.

HEMOLYTIC ANEMIA

In the US, hemolytic anemia continues to present an ongoing challenge to health care providers. Hemolytic anemia is defined as anemia occurring from lysis or destruction of RBCs.[29] Autoimmune hemolytic anemia (AIHA) is frequently idiopathic in nature.[30] Health care providers often manage anemia with the assumption of an iron deficiency cause.[31] AIHA accounts for one-half of all hemolytic anemias worldwide, with a 30% risk for developing this disease in patients with chronic lymphocytic leukemia (CLL), particularly those who have previously received purine analogues.[29]

Risk Factors and Classification

AIHA is an uncommon cause of anemia. Certain risk factors have been associated with hemolytic anemia (**Table 4**).[31]

The clinical presentation of AIHA varies depending on the severity and whether onset was abrupt or insidious. Hemolysis is defined as destruction or elimination RBCs from circulation before their 120-day life cycle. Hemolysis may present as either acute or chronic.[30] Severity of hemolysis is also a significant consideration on presentation. Patients presenting with a mild form of hemolysis may be asymptomatic; however, in more serious cases, the anemia can become life threatening. In most cases, the clinical presentation also reflects the underlying cause, as in SCA.[32]

Pathophysiology

Hemolysis is defined as premature destruction of erythrocytes. Autoimmune hemolysis occurs when antibodies in the immune system attack RBCs causing their

Table 4
Classifications of AIHA

Hereditary	Acquired
Membranopathies Enzymopathies Hemoglobinopathies	Immune Autoimmune • Warm antibody • Cold antibody
Metabolism G6PD deficiency	Alloimmune • Hemolytic transfusion reactions • Congenital hemolytic disease in newborns • Allografts (stem cell transplantation)
Hemoglobin Genetic abnormalities, ie., • Hb S • Hb C	Drug associated • Antimalarials • Sulfonamides • Analgesics, etc. Infections • Malaria, Clostridia Chemical agents • Industrial substances, benzene Secondary hemolysis • Associated with liver, renal disease, malignancy Signs and Symptoms • Fatigue • Pallor • Poor mental concentration • Shortness of breath, headaches • Bruising • Petechiae • Lightheadedness([33])

Abbreviations: G6PD, glucose-6-phosphte dehydrogenase; Hb, hemoglobin.

destruction bone marrow activity is unable to compensate for the loss of erythrocytes.[32] According to the US National Institutes of Health, multiple causes of RBC destruction exist.[33] The cause for autoimmune (RBC) destruction may be attributed to many factors, including abnormal hemoglobin S, immune destruction of erythrocytes, mechanical injury of RBCs, glucose-6-phosphte dehydrogenase (G6PD) deficiency, and intrinsic membrane defects.[34] However, 2 mechanisms of hemolysis are commonly described (**Table 5**)[26,35]:

1. Intravascular hemolysis: destruction of RBCs in circulation occurs with the release of cellular contents into plasma. Mechanical trauma occurs from a damaged endothelium, complement fixation, and activation on the cell surface, and infectious agents may result in direct breakdown of membrane and cell destruction. Evaluation of laboratory tests, including; serum bilirubin, reticulocyte count, haptoglobin and lactate dehydrogenase (LDH) levels may also assist in facilitating early indications of hemolysis.[36]
2. Extravascular hemolysis: removal and destruction of RBCs with membrane modifications by immune cells such as macrophages from the spleen and liver. A clear cause for AIHA remains unknown.[36]

Epidemiology

Hemolytic anemia represents 5% of all anemias; however, it is not known to be race specific and occurs with increased frequency throughout Africa, Asia, the Mediterranean, and the Middle East.[35–37] Schick characterizes hemolytic anemia as an X-linked recessive disorder primarily affecting women as predominant carriers.[36] In the United States, G6PD deficiency has been associated as a causative factor in hemolytic anemia, with 10% to 14% prevalence in African American men. Prevalence of the deficiency is correlated with the geographic distribution of malaria, theoretically proposing that carriers of G6PD deficiency may acquire partial defense against malaria.[37]

Diagnosis

Diagnosis is made primarily by diagnostic laboratory evaluation. The following are noted as pertinent laboratory tests: CBC, absolute reticulocyte count, direct and indirect bilirubin, serum LDH, direct antiglobin, bone marrow biopsy and aspirate, and a peripheral blood smear (**Table 6**).[38]

Table 5 Causes of hemolytic anemia	
Antibodies to RBC surface antigens	May be associated with malignancy, transfusions and drugs
Mechanical interference of RBC circulation	RBC destruction by antibodies
Infections	Such as malaria, babesiosis, and *Clostridium difficile*
G6PD deficiency	May be associated with infections, drugs, or ingestion of fava beans
Thalassemia and SCD	More prevalent in persons of African descent

Data from Dhaliwal G, Cornett PA, Tierney LM. Hemolytic anemia. Am Fam Physician 2004;69(11):2599–607.

Table 6
Pertinent diagnostic laboratory test for hemolysis

Laboratory Test	Explanation of Laboratory Values	Normal Range
Reticulocyte count (absolute)	Measures percentage of immature circulating RBCs in blood	0.5%–1.5 %
Direct and indirect Coombs test	Detection of antibodies that adhere to surface of RBCs	Coombs negative
Serum LDH	↑ LDH may symbolize hemolysis; nonspecific	313–618 µg/dL
Serum haptoglobin	Measures presence of hemolysis; active hemolysis indicated by values <20 mg/dL	30–200 mg/dL
Bone marrow biopsy and aspirate	Used to evaluate for fibrosis or immature cells	Normal cell production
Peripheral blood smear	Evaluates for presence of spherocytes/malignancy	Varies
CBC	Used to evaluate for anemia/ thrombocytopenia	12–16 g/dL

Data from Powers A, Silberstein LE. Autoimmune hemolytic anemia. In: Hoffman R, Benz EJ, Shattil SS, editors. Hematology: basic principles and practice. 5th edition. Philadelphia: Churchill Livingston Elsevier; 2008.

Treatment of Hemolysis

Management of hemolysis depends on the cause of the hemolysis. Several factors should be considered concerning treatment of AIHA, such as; age, medical history (whether previous history of autoimmune disease), overall health of the affected person, and life-expectancy may be a consideration. In physiologic causes, such as overactive immune system, immune suppressants may be indicated. It is also important to determine the goals of treatment, including; to reduce or stop destruction of RBCs, treat the underlying cause, and to restore or increase the RBC to a non-symptomatic level, if not able to restore to normal level.[39] Other treatments may include; an increase in folic acid and iron supplements, blood transfusions, and splenectomy (most effective among second-line therapy). Additionally, Rituxan (anti-CD20 antibody) is also useful as a second-line treatment for AIHA. In the presence of a warm antibody, steroids are the best primary treatment.[36,38,39]

SCA

SCA is a disease in which RBCs become distorted, forming a crescent shape that impedes blood flow through small blood vessels.[40] RBCs carry oxygen to body tissues and organs. SCA is characterized by the presence of hemoglobin S, which changes the shape of RBCs.[32,33] SCA is caused by a point mutation in the beta-globin chain of hemoglobin causing replacement of the hydrophilic amino acid valine. Loss of RBC elasticity decreases oxygen tension in the cell, promoting repeated episodes of sickling, ultimately causing irreparable damage to the cell membrane.[41]

SCD is viewed as a major health care and societal problem affecting millions worldwide.[40] SCD is the most common genetic disorder in the United States, with approximately 2000 infants born with the disease each year.[42]

Incidence/Prevalence

In the United States there are approximately 80,000 to 100,000 people living with SCD. It is commonly typified by intermittent, unanticipated episodes of severe pain with sudden onset leading to repeated emergency room visits.[43] SCD is most commonly found in people of African or Mediterranean descent; however, it is also seen in people from South and Central America, the Caribbean, and Middle Eastern regions.[32] In prevalent populations, mortality rate has been associated with frequency of sickle cell pain crises. Mortality has been associated with frequency of sickle cell pain crises.[40]

Causes/Risks Factors

SCA is caused by hemoglobin S. Risk factors are usually associated with familiar genetic involvement, because SCA is inherited from both parents (**Fig. 1**). Approximately 8% of African Americans are carriers because of the mutation in hemoglobin B causing structurally abnormal hemoglobin S. Symptoms start during early childhood and puberty.[33] Those at greater risk for developing SCD, include: descendants of Saharan Africa, Spanish-speaking areas of South American, the Caribbean; and Central America, Saudi Arabia, India, and Mediterranean countries.[35]

Signs and Symptoms

Acute and chronic pain is considered the hallmark of SCD, as in vaso-occlusive crisis pain. Bone pain, particularly in the long bones, is generally caused by marrow infarction. The bone marrow is unable to produce enough RBCs to keep up with the rate of destruction of RBCs, resulting in anemia that is usually hemolytic. In addition, the lifespan of RBCs is significantly shorter.[35] Symptoms associated with moderate to severe SCA, include: fatigue, shortness of breath, tachycardia, and paleness of skin and mucosal membranes. Jaundice may also occur, secondary to hemolysis of RBCs. In cases with occluded small blood vessels, priapism may result, as well as poor eyesight, mental confusion, and leg ulcers.[33,35,44] Adolescents may experience stunted growth and delayed puberty.

Acute chest syndrome (ACS) is a significant manifestation of SCD. In ACS, young children present with chest pain, fever, cough, tachypnea, leukocytosis, and pulmonary infiltrates throughout the upper lobes of the lungs.[44–47] However, adults usually present afebrile, with multilobar or lower lobe infiltrates, dyspnea, and severe chest pain.

Splenic sequestration may be a life-threatening complication of SCD requiring hospitalization. The cause of splenic sequestration is theorized to be that the spleen becomes engorged with trapped sickled cells, leading to splenic enlargement.[35] The sequestration process leads to associated symptoms, such as left-sided abdominal pain, weakness, excessive thirst, and tachypnea.

Pathophysiology

Hemoglobin S causes fragility of RBCs because of structural alteration of the RBC membrane. Sickled cells forfeit oxygen-carrying capacity, resulting in reduced oxygen delivery to body tissues and organs.[33] In addition, the process of sickling occurs, resulting in adherence to the walls of small blood vessels where hemolysis (cell destruction) occurs, thus triggering a pain crisis.

Treatment

Treatment is based on the clinical manifestations of SCD and is designed to manage and control symptoms. Hydroxyurea (Hydrea) is generally the drug of choice for the

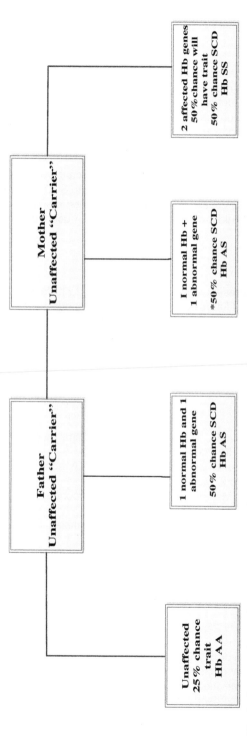

Fig. 1. Autosomal recessive genetic pattern of SCD. Hb, hemoglobin; Hb AA, hemoglobin unaffected; Hb AS, hemoglobin; Hb SS, sickle cell disease. (*Adapted from* Shiel WC. Sickle Cell Disease (Sickle Cell Anemia). http://www.nhlbi.nih.gov/health/topics.)

treatment of SCD.[33,35,40] Folic acid supplements are crucial because folic acid is required to make new RBCs. Other treatments that may be useful in SCA include antibiotics to prevent bacterial infections.

Pain Management

Because pain is the hallmark of SCD, pain management is essential.[40] In SCD, chronic pain may be attributed to many factors. However, vaso-occlusion of the microcirculation often leads to destruction of bones, joints, and visceral organs. The intensity of pain varies depending on the area most affected. Young children with this disease commonly experience abdominal pain.[33] Patients with SCD may experience numerous pain crises from vaso-occlusion. Management of acute SCD crisis generally occurs in hospital emergency centers.

Lanzkron and colleagues[43] (2010) noted the significant burden placed on emergency departments because of overuse by patients with SCD. Dunlop and Bennett[45] (2006) listed the following crises management strategies: opioids, nonsteroidals, hydration (ie, intravenous fluids, oral fluid intake), oxygen use, vitamins (ie, folic acid), and vaccines.

SUMMARY

In summary, anemias present significant expense and challenges to the US health care system. The focus of future research is primarily genetic research and associated risk factors that predispose patients to anemias. It is of vital importance for health care providers to be aware of the various types of anemia, as well as the recommended management strategies. Various types of anemias, including iron and B_{12}, hemolytic anemia, SCA, and SCD, are discussed in this article with appropriate evidence-based management strategies. Research of various aspects of anemia is ongoing.

REFERENCES

1. Beutler E, Lichtman MA, Coller BS, et al. Williams hematology. 6th edition. New York: McGraw-Hill; 2001.
2. Clinical approach to anemia. In: Hillman RS, Ault KA, editors. Hematology in clinical practice. New York: McGraw-Hill; 2001. p. 29.
3. Zingraff J, Drüeke T, Marie P, et al. Anemia and secondary hyperparathyroidism. Arch Intern Med 1978;138(11):1650.
4. Nathan DG, Oski FA. Hematology of infancy and childhood. 4th edition. Philadelphia: WB Saunders; 1993. p. 352.
5. Bull BS, Breton-Gorius J. Morphology of the erythron. In: Beutler E, Lichtman MA, Coller BS, editors. Williams hematology. 5th edition. New York: McGraw-Hill; 1995. p. 349.
6. Hoffbrand V, Provan D. ABC of clinical haematology. Macrocytic anaemias. BMJ 1997;314(7078):430.
7. Anand IS. Pathophysiology of anemia in heart failure. Heart Fail Clin 2010;6(3):279–88.
8. Strobach RS, Anderson SK, Doll DC, et al. The value of the physical examination in the diagnosis of anemia. Arch Intern Med 1988;148(4):831–2.
9. World Health Organization. Nutritional anaemias: report of a WHO scientific group. Geneva (Switzerland): World Health Organization; 1968.
10. Johnson-Wimbley TD, Graham D. Diagnosis and management of iron deficiency anemia in the 21st century. Therap Adv Gastroenterol 2011;4(3):177–84.

11. Clark SF. Iron deficiency anemia: diagnosis and management. Curr Opin Gastroenterol 2009;25:122–8.
12. Looker AD, Dallman PR, Carroll MD. Prevalence of iron deficiency in the united states. JAMA 1997;277:973–6.
13. Gisbert JP, Gomollon F. A guide to diagnosis of iron deficiency and iron deficiency anemia in digestive diseases. World J Gastroenterol 2009;15(37): 4638–43.
14. Hillman RS, Henderson PA. Control of marrow production by the level of iron supply. J Clin Invest 1969;48:454–60.
15. Cook JD, Flowers CH, Skikne BS. The quantitative assessment of body iron. Blood 2003;101:3359.
16. Howell JT, Monto RW. Syndrome of anemia, dysphagia and glossitis (Plummer Vinson syndrome). N Engl J Med 1953;249:1009.
17. Crosby WH. Whatever became of chlorosis? JAMA 1987;257:2799.
18. Reynolds RD, Binder HJ, Miller M, et al. Pagophagia and iron deficiency anemia. Ann Intern Med 1968;69:435.
19. Rector WG. Pica: its frequency and significance in patients with iron-deficiency anemia due to chronic gastrointestinal blood loss. J Gen Intern Med 1989;4:512.
20. Fairbanks VF. Laboratory testing for iron status. Hosp Pract 1990;26:17.
21. Guyatt GH, Oxman AD, Ali M, et al. Laboratory diagnosis of iron-deficiency anemia: an overview. J Gen Intern Med 1992;7(2):145.
22. Recommendations to prevent and control iron deficiency in the United States. Centers for Disease Control and Prevention (CDC). MMWR Recomm Rep 1998; 47:1–29.
23. National Institutes of Health (NIH). Dietary supplement fact sheet: iron. Bethesda (MD): Office of Dietary Supplements, National Institutes of Health; 2010. Available at: http://ods.od.nih.gov/factsheets/iron/. Accessed January 15, 2013.
24. Obrley MJ, Yang DT. Laboratory testing for cobalamin deficiency in megaloblastic anemia. Am J Hematol 2013;88(6):522–6. Available at: http://wileyonlinelibrary.com/cgi-bin/jhome/35105. Published online March 5, 2013.
25. Lechner K, Godinger M, Grisold W, et al. Vitamin B12 deficiency: new data on an old theme. Wien Klin Wochenschr 2005;117(17):579–91.
26. Stabler SP. Vitamin B12 deficiency. N Engl J Med 2013;368:149–60. Available at: http://www.nejm.org/doi/full/10.1056/NEJMcp1113996. Accessed January 15, 2013.
27. Monsen AL, Ueland PM. Homocysteine and methylmalonic acid in diagnosis and risk assessment from infancy to adolescence. Am J Clin Nutr 2003;78(1): 7–21.
28. MedlinePlus. Anemia-B12 deficiency. MedlinePlus; 2012. Available at: http://www.nlm.nih.gov/medlineplus/ency/article/000574.htm. Accessed January 15, 2013.
29. Chen Y, Zieve D. Hemolytic anemia. 2012. Available at: http://www.ncbi.nlm.gov/pubmedhealth/PMH0001597/. Accessed January 8, 2013.
30. Dhaliwal G, Cornett PA, Tierney LM. Hemolytic anemia. Am Fam Physician 2004; 69(11):2599–607.
31. American Society of Hematology. Available at: www.asheducationbook.hematologylibrary.org. Accessed May 7, 2013.
32. National Center for Biotechnology Information. Available at: http://www.ncbi.nih.gov/pubmedhealth/PMH0001554/?report. Accessed April 26, 2013.
33. National Institute of Health. Available at: http://www.nih.gov. Accessed December 5, 2012.

34. Gehrs BB, Friedberg RC. Autoimmune hemolytic anemia. Am J Hematol 2002; 69(4):258–71.
35. Center for Disease Control. 2012. Available at: http://www.cdc.gov/ncbddd/ sicklecell/treatments.html. Accessed November 15, 2012.
36. Schick P. Hemolytic anemia. 2013. Available at: http://www.medscape.com. Accessed January 4, 2013.
37. Frank J, Maj MC. Diagnosis and management of G6PD deficiency. Am Fam Physician 2005;72(7):1277–82.
38. Schrier S, Mentzer WC, Landaw SA, editors. Approach to diagnosis of hemolytic anemia in the adult. 2013. Available at: www.uptodateonline.com.
39. Lechner K, Jager Ulrich. How I treat autoimmune hemolytic anemias in adults. Blood 2010;116(11):1831–8.
40. Taylor LV, Stotts NA, Humphreys J, et al. A review of the literature on the multiple dimensions of chronic pain in adults with sickle cell disease. J Pain Symptom Manage 2010;40(3):416–35. http://dx.doi.org/10.1016/j.jpainsymman.2009.12.027.
41. Valavi E, Ansari MA, Zandiark K. How to reach rapid diagnosis in sickle cell disease. Iran J Pediatr 2010;20(1):61–74.
42. Kavanagh PL, Sprinz PG, Vinci SR, et al. Management of children with sickle cell disease: a comprehensive review of the literature. Pediatrics 2011;128(6): e1552–74.
43. Lanzkron S, Caroll CP, Haywood C. The burden of emergency department use for sickle-cell disease: an analysis of the national emergency department sample database. Am J Hematol 2010;85(10):797–9.
44. Maakaron JE, Besa EC, editors. Sickle cell anemia. 2013. Available at: http:// www.emedicine.medscape.com/article/205926-overview. Accessed May 7, 2013.
45. Dunlop RJ, Bennett KC. Pain management for sickle cell disease. Cochrane Database Syst Rev 2006;(2). CD003350. Available at: www.ncbi.nlm.nih.gov/ pubmed/16625580. Accessed January 4, 2013.
46. Ballas SK. Sickle cell anaemia: progress in pathogenesis and treatment. Drugs 2002;62(8):1143–72.
47. Bunn HF. Approach to the anemias. In: Goldman L, Scafer AI, editors. 24th edition. Philadelphia: Saunders Elsevier; 2011.

Thrombocytopenia

Edythe M. (Lyn) Greenberg, PhD, RN, FNP-BC*,
Elizabeth S. (Sue) Kaled, MS, RN, NP-C, FNP-BC

KEYWORDS

- Thrombocytopenia • Bleeding • Platelets

KEY POINTS

- Thrombocytopenia is a platelet count less than 150,000/μL.
- Thrombocytopenia is caused by decreased platelet production, sequestration of platelets, or increased destruction of platelets.
- Thrombocytopenia has many causes, including infections, cancer, liver disease, autoimmune disorders, disseminated intravascular coagulation, pregnancy, medications, and coagulation disorders.
- Treatment of thrombocytopenia is determined by the underlying cause.

INTRODUCTION

Platelets are the first line of defense against bleeding. They are made by the megakaryocytes in the bone marrow. The bone marrow microenvironment regulates the proliferation, differentiation, and platelet budding of the megakaryocytes. Their production is regulated by cytokines and chemokines. Thrombopoietin, which is produced primarily in the liver, is the most potent stimulator of thrombopoiesis, which is the process of making new platelets. It promotes both the proliferation of megakaryocyte (platelet) progenitors and the maturation of the megakaryocytes. On maturation, they generate and release new platelets into the circulation.[1,2] Platelets live for approximately 7 to 10 days. However, their life span may be shortened because of increased platelet destruction. The number of circulating platelets is determined by platelet production or number of platelets entering the circulation, and platelet destruction under steady-state conditions.[1]

Platelets are part of the extrinsic clotting pathway. The normal vascular endothelium is smooth and secretes nitric oxide, which prevents platelets from adhering. When a

Relationship: Neither E.S. (Sue) Kaled nor E.M. (Lyn) Greenberg has any direct financial interest with a commercial company.
Department of Leukemia, MD Anderson Cancer Center, 1515 Holcombe Boulevard, Houston, TX 77030, USA
* Corresponding author.
E-mail address: emgreenberg@mdanderson.edu

disruption occurs in the vascular endothelium, platelets adhere to the vascular lining. They release nucleotides, adhesive proteins, growth factors, and procoagulants, which cause platelet aggregation and blood clot formation, and attract other platelets to the site of injury. The platelet plug is strengthened by the fibrin mesh that forms from the intrinsic clotting cascade.[1,3] The platelet plug is a reason why hemophiliacs do not exsanguinate.[1]

Thrombocytopenia is defined as a platelet count less than 150,000/μL. It is considered to be mild when the platelet count is between 70,000 and 150,000/μL, and severe if less than 20,000/μL. Most individuals are asymptomatic if the platelet count is 50,000/μL or greater. Surgical procedures may be performed when the platelet count is 50,000/μL or greater.[4] Bleeding from minimal trauma may occur with a platelet count of 30,000/μL or less, and spontaneous bleeding may occur when the platelet count is less than 10,000/μL.[4] Spontaneous bleeding may occur in the mucosa, skin, lungs, gastrointestinal tract, central nervous system, and genitourinary tract.[4]

Thrombocytopenia can occur from a decreased bone marrow production, increased destruction of platelets, and sequestration.[1,4] This article discusses the evaluation and management of common causes of thrombocytopenia.

EVALUATION OF THROMBOCYTOPENIA
History

The history of a patient's present illness includes any events that may be associated with thrombocytopenia, although often it is an incidental finding. The past medical history should include any previous illnesses and recent infections, malignancies (eg, myelodysplastic syndrome, leukemia, lymphoma, aplastic anemia), recent travel (which may suggest dengue fever, malaria, rickettsial infections, possible tick bite), recent new medications, organ transplant, transfusion history, alcohol or drug use, recent hospitalizations, immunizations, high-risk behaviors, over-the-counter medications/herbs, autoimmune disorders, and pregnancy. Patients should be asked about any family history of bleeding disorders and whether they have experienced any bleeding episodes (eg, nosebleeds, easy bruising, heavy menses in a woman of childbearing age, prolonged bleeding after procedures, bleeding gums, blood in sputum, blood in urine, melena), fever, rashes, pain, headache, or vision changes.[4–6] Patients who have a central venous catheter should be asked if they are flushing with normal saline or heparin.

Physical Examination

The physical examination should make note of bleeding, bruising (petechiae, purpura, ecchymosis), enlarged liver or spleen, and ischemic limb or skin necrosis associated with heparin-induced thrombocytopenia.[6] A stool for occult blood should be obtained to evaluate for gastrointestinal/rectal bleeding. A fundoscopic examination can provide evidence of central nervous system bleeding if hemorrhages are present. Any areas of bruising should be marked to note the bleeding pattern. The patient should be evaluated for painful, swollen joints, and any epistaxis, hematuria, blood in sputum, oozing from the gums, alterations in mental status, and abdominal tenderness and distention should be noted.[5,6]

Laboratory Data

When evaluating the complete blood cell count with differential, all 3 cell lineages (white blood cells, red blood cells/hemoglobin, and platelets) are evaluated. Rapid evaluation and treatment are indicated when peripheral blood blasts are seen, because this indicates an acute leukemia. Red blood cell fragmentation is associated with thrombotic microangiography,[6] and also requires an astute evaluation. If disseminated intravascular coagulation (DIC) is suspected, then a D-dimer and coagulation studies are obtained in addition to the platelet count.

A pseudothrombocytopenia can occur with platelet clumping. Pseudothrombocytopenia accounts for approximately 15% to 30% of all isolated cases of thrombocytopenia.[7] Normally, platelet count measurements using electronic particle counters are more accurate and less expensive than manual techniques. Unfortunately, underestimation of platelets occurs because of in vitro platelet clumping or platelet adherence to leukocytes, which is not detected by the electronic particle counters, and therefore the reports produced are inaccurate. Approximately 0.1% of the population has an ethylene diamine tetra-acetic acid–dependent platelet-agglutinating antibody. This antibody causes the platelets to clump on the prepared slides. In vivo, the platelet counts are normal.[8] If pseudothrombocytopenia occurs, a microscopic examination for platelet clumping and a repeat platelet count should be repeated using a different anticoagulant, such as heparin or sodium citrate, as the anticoagulant.[9]

DECREASED PLATELET PRODUCTION
Viral Infections

Viral infections such as the human immunodeficiency virus (HIV), hepatitis B, hepatitis C, Epstein-Barr, cytomegalovirus, parvovirus B19, varicella-zoster, rubella, and mumps are associated with thrombocytopenia because of bone marrow suppression.[4,5] HIV infections may present with an initial decrease in the platelet count, but it is more prevalent with nontreated HIV infections. The cause is a combination of shortened platelet life span, splenic sequestration, and HIV-infected megakaryocytes, therefore decreasing the ability to produce platelets.[7,10] As hepatitis C advances, the thrombocytopenia worsens and can become multifocal from a decreased thrombopoietin production from the liver, bone marrow inhibition, and an autoimmune component.[11] In a self-limited viral illness such as H1N1, the platelet counts usually recover.[4]

Bacterial, Viral, and Rickettsial Infections

Infections such as malaria and tuberculosis affect the platelet count through a combined effect of immune-mediated destruction, splenic sequestration, and shortened platelet survival time.[12] Tuberculosis can present with a granulomatosis infiltration of the bone marrow, which can cause thrombocytopenia, or in rare cases immune thrombocytopenia purpura (ITP), in addition to other cytopenias. Immune presentation includes elevated platelet associated immunoglobulin G (IgG) levels.[13] Rickettsial infections such as Rocky Mountain spotted fever and Lyme disease may have a transient thrombocytopenia.[4]

Bone Marrow Suppression and Malignancies

Thrombocytopenia occurs with primary neoplastic disorders of the bone marrow, including myeloid disorders such as acute myeloid leukemia, myelodysplastic syndrome, myeloproliferative syndromes, and paroxysmal nocturnal hemoglobinuria. Lymphoid malignancies, such as acute lymphoid leukemia, hairy cell leukemia, chronic lymphoid leukemias, non-Hodgkin lymphoma, T-cell malignancies, multiple myeloma, and Waldenström macroglobulinemia may also present with a thrombocytopenia. Infiltration of the bone marrow by fibrotic tissue, myelofibrosis, and nonhematologic malignancies, such as prostate and breast cancer, can also cause thrombocytopenia.[4]

Radiotherapy and high-dose chemotherapy can cause thrombocytopenia. Myelo-dysplastic syndrome (MDS) is often a secondary result of previous radiotherapy and high-dose chemotherapy. Bone marrow suppression may occur up to 5 years after treatment.[7] Individuals who are treated for hematologic malignancies receive frequent platelet transfusions. They can become platelet-refractory from an autoimmune response to the HLAs on leukocytes in the transfused platelets. Individuals who are refractory to platelets can be managed with single donor platelet transfusions, trans-fusions of HLA platelets, or transfusing the platelets over a longer period. Aplastic ane-mia is associated with anemia, neutropenia, and thrombocytopenia from bone marrow failure.[1]

Liver Disease and Chronic Alcohol Abuse

Thrombocytopenia occurs in chronic liver disease, such as drug-induced liver dis-ease, infectious hepatitis, nonalcoholic liver disease, and metabolic disorders.[4] Thrombocytopenia in the presence of alcohol abuse is related to cirrhosis of the liver, hypersplenism, and folic acid deficiency. Thrombocytopenia in this instance is a com-bination of a decreased production of thrombopoietin from the liver and sequestration of platelets in the spleen. Thrombocytopenia may also be higher in chronic alcoholism associated with a megaloblastic anemia from vitamin B_{12} and folic acid deficiencies.[1] However, alcohol-induced thrombocytopenia can occur in the absence of liver dis-ease or nutrient deficiency. When the alcohol consumption is stopped, the platelet count gradually increases and recovers normal counts in 7 to 10 days.[14] Treatment in-cludes advising the patient to discontinue alcohol ingestion and prescribing nutri-tional/vitamin replacement.[4]

SEQUESTRATION

Monocytes from the bone marrow migrate to different parts of the body to help protect the organism. These monocytes become part of the reticuloendothelial system. In the spleen, these cells are called *reticular cells*. Splenic reticular cells primarily function to remove the senescent cells from circulation and provide phagocytic cells for both in-flammatory and immune responses. Occasionally, platelets are shifted into the spleen, and the platelet count looks low despite normal or increased total numbers. The retic-ular cells may be triggered to sense normal platelets as abnormal or foreign, and cull them from the circulation. This process can occur with portal hypertension, sarcoid-osis, lymphomas, Gaucher disease, Felty syndrome, myelofibrosis, and chronic lym-phocytic leukemia (CLL).[15]

INCREASED DESTRUCTION OF PLATELETS
Autoimmune Syndromes

ITP, also known as *idiopathic thrombocytopenic purpura*, is an autoimmune disorder resulting in a low platelet count from increased destruction of platelets or impaired thrombopoiesis by antiplatelet antibodies. A bone marrow study may be ordered to evaluate the thrombocytopenia. The bone marrow study may report either a normal or an increased number of megakaryocytes.[1] The hemoglobin and hematocrit may be normal unless an autoimmune hemolytic anemia is also present.[1,4]

Secondary immune thrombocytopenia is associated with autoimmune disorders, such as systemic lupus erythematosus, Grave disease, and sarcoidosis.[4] Individuals with CLL may initially present with an autoimmune thrombocytopenia. The risk of bleeding is determined by the platelet count. Asymptomatic individuals may be managed with observation and frequent monitoring. Symptomatic immune-mediated

ITP is treated with oral steroids, intravenous IgG, the monoclonal antibody rituximab (Rituxan), or a splenectomy.[1,4] A newer treatment option is the use of thrombopoietin mimetic drugs, such as eltrombopag (Promacta) and romiplostim (Nplate). Alternative treatments for refractory autoimmune thrombocytopenia include vinca alkaloids (vincristine, vinblastine), cyclophosphamide (Cytoxan), azathioprine, and danazol.[1]

Pulmonary Emboli

Antiphospholipid syndrome is associated with a recent fetal loss. Thrombocytopenia with a pulmonary embolism is an autoimmune phenomenon. Another cause of pulmonary emboli with thrombocytopenia is heparin-induced thrombocytopenia (HIT), also associated with antibodies as a result of the heparin.[16–18]

DIC

DIC is a dysregulation of the clotting mechanisms that leads to clotting in the microcirculation and bleeding. It can be associated with severe infection/sepsis, severe trauma, pregnancy, liver disease, transplant rejection, snake bites, ABO-incompatible blood transfusions, malignancies (eg, acute promyelocytic leukemia), and vascular abnormalities.[6,19] It is diagnosed based on the clinical presentation supported by laboratory findings, including a low platelet count, a prolonged partial thromboplastin time, a prolonged prothrombin time, and elevated levels of D-dimer and fibrin degradation products. If available, a reduction in the antithrombin and protein C levels may be significant, but a single determination is not sufficient to make the diagnosis of DIC. Fibrinogen levels are not very useful unless the case of DIC is severe. Primary treatment consists of treating the underlying cause. Platelet transfusions, cryoprecipitate, and fresh frozen plasma are not administered unless the patient is actively bleeding. Because of the high risk of venous thromboembolic phenomena, anticoagulants such as heparin, low-molecular-weight heparin, and mechanical methods, such as graded compression stockings and intermittent pneumatic leg compression, are frequently used to treat DIC.[19]

DRUG-INDUCED THROMBOCYTOPENIA

Many medications have been associated with drug-induced thrombocytopenia. The goal of management is to remove the offending medication before any clinically significant bleeding or, in the case of heparin, thrombosis occurs. The main mechanisms for drug-induced thrombocytopenia are an immune-mediated destruction and impaired platelet production. Unfortunately, most instances of drug-induced thrombocytopenia occur in individuals who are taking multiple agents to control other medical conditions. Therefore, the causative medication may be difficult to identify.[16]

Impaired platelet production is most frequently caused by chemotherapeutic agents in a dose-dependent, inverse manner. In other words, high-dose chemotherapy can lower the platelets count because it suppresses the bone marrow. Other medications, such as chloramphenicol, phenylbutazone, and gold, cause bone marrow suppression, but only in susceptible people. Valproic acid has a dose-dependent pattern of thrombocytopenia. Ganciclovir is also directly mylosuppressive.[16,17]

Many drugs are capable of causing antibody-mediated thrombocytopenia. Some drugs bind to platelet membrane glycoproteins, which stimulate production of antibodies that interact with antigens on the platelets, resulting in a thrombocytopenia.[1] Quinidine, quinine, and sulfonamides can produce a thrombocytopenia from this type of antibody-antigen reaction. When the drug is discontinued, the platelet count recovers.[1] A complete list of medications that induce thrombocytopenia can be found at www.ouhsc.edu/platelets.

HIT typically begins within a week of starting heparin and is caused by antibodies that recognize the complex formed between heparin and platelet factor 4 (PF4). This condition evolves into an environment conducive to thrombosis formation, with deep vein thrombosis, pulmonary embolism, stroke, and myocardial infarction being the most common complications.[4,16–18] Treatment is to discontinue the heparin, and use a nonheparin anticoagulant such as a thrombin inhibitor, including lepirudin (Refludan) or argatroban (Argatroban).[20] Warfarin should not be administered until the platelet count has recovered, because it may lead to microvascular thrombosis in patients with HIT. Vitamin K can be administered if warfarin was started as an anticoagulant.[21]

UREMIA

Patients with uremia, especially those undergoing dialysis, may develop thrombocytopenia. The kidneys also produce thrombopoietin, although to a lesser degree than the liver. Decreased thrombopoietin production can lead to decreased platelet production.[2] During hemodialysis, additional platelet destruction may occur because of platelet consumption in the dialyzer membrane.[22]

PREGNANCY
Gestational Thrombocytopenia

Thrombocytopenia is the second most common hematologic disorder during pregnancy.[1] Gestational thrombocytopenia is a benign disorder caused by the expanded plasma volume in a woman with no history of thrombocytopenia or fetal thrombocytopenia.[4] However, other causes of thrombocytopenia must be eliminated before determining that the thrombocytopenia is benign. Gestational thrombocytopenia is not associated with increased bleeding or ill effects on the fetus, and usually resolves spontaneously after the delivery. Autoimmune thrombocytopenia may be exacerbated by pregnancy. No blood test exists to determine whether thrombocytopenia during pregnancy is related to normal gestational changes or autoimmune thrombocytopenia. In women who have a history of autoimmune thrombocytopenia, this diagnosis if favored.[1]

HELLP Syndrome

Thrombocytopenia can also occur in preeclampsia, eclampsia, and HELLP syndrome. HELLP syndrome is defined by hemolysis, elevated liver enzymes (lactate dehydrogenase, aspartate aminotransferase), and a low platelet count.[1,23,24] HELLP syndrome may be a variant of preeclampsia or can occur on its own in association with preeclampsia.[24] Although the cause of HELLP syndrome is unknown, risk factors include a previous pregnancy with HELLP syndrome, pregnancy-induced hypertension, age older than 25 years, Caucasian race, and multiparity.[23,24] Any pregnant woman who is at least 20 weeks pregnant, and presents with a headache, changes in vision, right upper quadrant abdominal pain, nausea and vomiting, fatigue/malaise, proteinuria, edema, and hypertension should be evaluated for preeclampsia and HELLP syndrome.[4,23,24]

If HELLP syndrome is suspected, a complete blood cell count with differential, urinalysis, a coagulation panel, and liver function tests should be ordered. The hematocrit may be normal or low. Elevated liver function tests and a positive D-dimer may be predictive of women who may develop HELLP syndrome. The coagulation studies will be normal unless DIC is present.[24]

HELLP syndrome usually subsides within 2 to 3 days after delivery.[23] The best treatment for HELLP syndrome, eclampsia, and preeclampsia is administering magnesium sulfate and delivering the fetus.[1,4] In severe HELLP syndrome, plasma exchange is the treatment if the fetus is less than 34 weeks' gestation or no improvement occurs in the first week postpartum.[1] Other supportive measures include bed rest, antihypertensive medications, corticosteroids, fetal monitoring, and platelet transfusions. Complications of HELLP syndrome include placenta abruption, pulmonary edema, DIC, adult respiratory distress syndrome, acute renal failure, ruptured liver hematoma, intrauterine growth restriction, infant respiratory distress, and complications of blood/platelet transfusions.[23]

OTHER CONSIDERATIONS

Life-threatening emergencies associated with thrombocytopenia during pregnancy include DIC, which may occur with sepsis and placenta abruption, and thrombotic thrombocytopenic purpura.[4] In the intensive care unit, when evaluating thrombocytopenia, one should consider DIC; infection/sepsis; massive blood transfusions; the use of heparin; cardiopulmonary resuscitation; cardiopulmonary bypass; adult respiratory distress syndrome; pulmonary embolism; solid organ allograft rejection; and medications.[5] Thrombocytopenia may be the result of a cardiopulmonary bypass, caused by mechanical destruction of the platelets, hemodilution in the bypass circuit, medications, intra-aortic balloon pumping, and posttransfusion purpura.[6]

SUMMARY

Thrombocytopenia has multiple causes, and its treatment is tailored to the underlying disease process. Nurses play an important role in the management of thrombocytopenia. An astute nursing assessment enables rapid intervention when life-threatening bleeding is present from the thrombocytopenia. The nursing history may identify any medications, infections, or health behaviors that are causing the thrombocytopenia. As new medications, such as thrombopoietin mimetics, are developed for thrombocytopenia related to marrow dysfunction, the nurse will become a primary educational resource. Thrombocytopenia is a health issue in which nursing has the potential to make an impact.

REFERENCES

1. Konkle B. Disorders of platelets and vessel wall. In: Longo DL, Fauci AS, Kasper DL, et al, editors. Harrison's principles of internal medicine, vol. 1, 18th edition. New York: McGraw Hill Medical; 2012. p. 965–73.
2. Qian S, Fu F, Li W, et al. Primary role of the liver in thrombopoietin production shown by tissue-specific knockout. Blood 1998;92:2189–91.
3. Nabili ST. Thrombocytopenia. Available at: http://www.medicinenet.com/thrombocytopenia_low_platelet_count/article.htm. Accessed March 15, 2013.
4. Gauer RL, Braun MM. Thrombocytopenia. Am Fam Physician 2012;85:612–22.
5. Thiagarajan P, Besa EC. Platelet disorders overview of platelet disorders. Available at: http://emedicine.medscape.com/article/201722-overview. Accessed March 22, 2013.
6. Stasi R. How to approach thrombocytopenia. Available at: http://asheducationbook.hematologylibrary.org. Accessed March 15, 2013.
7. Diz-Kucukkaya R, Chen J, Gedis A, et al. Thrombocytopenia. In: Kaushansky K, Lichtman MA, Beutler E, et al, editors. Williams hematology. 8th edition. New York: McGraw Hill Medical; 2010. p. 1431–81.

8. Casonato A, Bertomoro A, Pontara E, et al. EDTA dependent pseudothrombocytopenia caused by antibodies against the cytoadhesive receptor of platelet gpIIB-IIIA. J Clin Pathol 1994;47:625–30.
9. Chia J, Hsia CC. Pseudothrombocytopenia. Blood 2011;117(16):4168.
10. Cole JL, Marzec UM, Gunthel CJ, et al. Ineffective platelet production in thrombocytopenic human immunodeficiency virus-infected patients. Blood 1998;91: 3239–46.
11. Olariu M, Olariu C, Olteanu D. Thrombocytopenia in chronic hepatitis C. J Gastrointestin Liver Dis 2010;19:381–5.
12. Nithish B, Vikram G, Hariprasad S. Thrombocytopenia in malaria: a clinical study. Biomedical Research 2011;22:489–91.
13. Tsuro K, Kojima H, Mitoro A, et al. Immune thrombocytopenia purpura associated with pulmonary tuberculosis. Intern Med 2006;22:489–91.
14. Ballard H. Hematologic complications of alcoholism. Alcohol Health Res World 1997;21:42–52.
15. Kuwana M, Okazaki Y, Ikeda Y. Splenic macrophages maintain the anti-platelet autoimmune response via uptake of opsonized platelets in patients with immune thrombocytopenic purpura. J Thromb Haemost 2009;7:322–9.
16. Wazny L, Ariano R. Evaluation and management of drug-induced thrombocytopenia in the acutely ill patient. Pharmacotherapy 2000;20:292–307.
17. George J, Aster R. Drug-induced thrombocytopenia: pathogenesis, evaluation, and management. Hematology 2009;7:911–8.
18. Greinacher A, Eichler P, Lubenow N, et al. Drug-induced and drug dependent immune thrombocytopenias. Rev Clin Exp Hematol 2001;5:166–200.
19. Levi M, Toh CH, Thachil J, et al. Guidelines for the diagnosis and management of disseminated intravascular coagulation. Br J Haematol 2009;145:24–33.
20. Pravinkumar E, Webster NR. HIT/HITT and alternative anticoagulation: Current concepts. Br J Anaesth 2003;90:675–85.
21. Baroletti SA, Goldhaber SZ. Heparin-induced thrombocytopenia. Available at: http://circ.ahajournals.org. Accessed March 15, 2013.
22. Dangirdas J, Bernardo A. Hemodialysis effect on platelet count and function and hemodialysis-associated thrombocytopenia. Kidney Int 2012;82:147–57.
23. HELLP syndrome. American Pregnancy Association Web site. Available at: http://americanpregnancy.org/pregnancycomplications/hellpsyndrome.html. Accessed March 13, 2013.
24. Padden MO. HELLP syndrome: recognition and perinatal management. Am Fam Physician 1999;60:829–36.

Hemostasis, Coagulation Abnormalities, and Liver Disease

Carole L. Mackavey, RN, MSN, FNP-C[a],*,
Robert Hanks, PhD, FNP-C, RNC[b]

KEYWORDS

- Hemostasis • Coagulation abnormalities • Liver disease • Procoagulants
- Anticoagulants • Fibrinolysis

KEY POINTS

- Liver disease is frequently complicated by bleeding and thrombic diathesis.
- Activated partial thromboplastin time and prothrombin time are poor predictors of thrombic or bleeding risk.
- Detecting bleeding diathesis involves vigilance and close observation.

INTRODUCTION

The bleeding diathesis associated with coagulopathy present in patients with liver disease is a common clinical concern. Approximately 70% of the patients with chronic liver disease (CLD) will experience varices and 50% to 72% will experience bleeding.[1,2] The role of the liver undergoes considerable change during hemostasis, in the presence of both acute and chronic disease. Coagulopathy in liver disease is a complex feedback mechanism striving to maintain a balance between platelets, coagulation factors, and fibrinolysis. The prevalence of CLD has gradually increased over the past few decades. Between 1988 and 1994, the prevalence was 11.78%. Between 1999 and 2004, it climbed to 15.66%. Finally, between 2005 and 2008, it slightly declined to 14.78%.[1] CLD includes cirrhosis, hepatitis B and C, and other viruses, as well as nonalcoholic fatty liver disease (NAFLD).[1] These rates are relatively stable, as is the rate of 35% for hepatitis-associated liver disease. However, the prevalence of NAFLD, during the same period, increased from 5.51% to 9.84% and 11.01%, consecutively.[1] From 1988 to 1994, NAFLD accounted for 46.8% of chronic liver

Disclosure: The authors have identified no professional of financial affiliation for themselves or their spouse or partner.
[a] University of Texas Health Science Center at Houston, Houston, TX, USA; [b] Graduate Nurse Education Demonstration Project, School of Nursing, University of Texas Health Science Center at Houston, Houston, TX, USA
* Corresponding author.
E-mail address: c.mackavey@att.net

cases. From 1994 to 2004, its prevalence increased to 62.84% and, from 2005 to 2008, to 75.1%. This coincides with the increased rate of obesity and metabolic syndrome.[1]

PATHOPHYSIOLOGY

Coagulopathy in liver disease is linked to liver function and the decreased production of many of the coagulation-related proteins. Hepatic parenchymal cells are responsible for the formation of fibrinogen, factors II, V, VII, IX, XI, XII, and XIII. The decreased production of these blood proteins significantly affects hemostasis, increasing the possibility of bleeding events. With liver disease, these proteins normally have a very short half-life (**Fig. 1**), degrading so quickly that the liver is unable to keep up with the production needs of the body. The degradation of the proteins, which is one of the first signs of liver disease, results in the elevation of prothrombin time (PT) and the international normalized ratio (INR). Because of the alteration in liver function, bleeding is a major clinical concern in patients with liver disease.[2]

NORMAL CLOTTING CASCADE

Hemostasis is the result of a series of complex enzymatic reactions occurring simultaneously through the extrinsic pathway (also known as the tissue factor [TF] pathway) and the intrinsic pathway (also known as the contact activation pathway). Platelets and fibrin are the two major blood components needed for repair when an injury to the blood vessel wall occurs. The endothelial layer of the blood vessel prevents the accumulation of platelets and fibrin. When an injury occurs to the vessel wall, exposing the subendothelial layer, bleeding begins and a hemostatic plug develops. This process results in primary hemostasis (**Fig. 2**).[3–6]

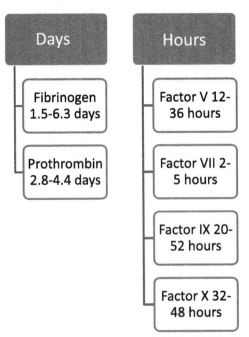

Fig. 1. Half-life of clotting factors. (*Data from* Munoz SJ, Stravitz RT, Gabriel DA. Coagulopathy of acute liver failure. Clin Liver Dis 2009;13(1):95–107.)

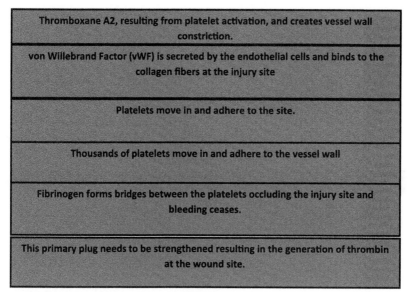

Fig. 2. Primary hemostasis. (*Data from* Refs.[3–6])

THE CLOTTING CASCADE

The initiation of the clotting cascade (**Fig. 3**)[3–6] begins when free TF is released from subendothelial stores and platelets start the coagulation cascade with its interaction with activated (a) factor VII. The combination of TF and factor VIIa convert factor X to factor Xa. TF and factor VIIa also convert factor IX to factor IXa. However, further activation of factor Xa is inhibited by the activate TF (aTF) pathway inhibitor. By this time, there has been enough thrombin made by factor Xa to activate factors VIII and V. Factor VIII then accelerates the activation of factor X by factor IXa. Factor VIIIa increases the ability of factor IXa to convert factor X to factor Xa thousands of times. Factor V amplifies the activation of prothrombin by factor Xa. Factor Xa along with factor Va and calcium creates the conversion of prothrombin to thrombin. Thrombin with thrombomodulin then acts on fibrinogen to form fibrin. The result is fibrin and wound healing. The fibrin seals the plug and stabilizes the clot. During the next 7 to 10 days, the fibrin dissolves and wound healing is completed.[3–6]

ANTICOAGULANTS: PROTEIN C AND PROTEIN S

The protein C pathway coexists and interacts with the common pathway and serves as a major system for controlling thrombosis, limiting inflammatory responses, and potentially decreasing endothelial cell apoptosis in response to inflammatory cytokines and ischemia. The essential components of the pathway involve thrombin, thrombomodulin, the endothelial cell protein C receptor (EPCR), protein C, and protein S.[7] The protein C pathway also plays a role in maintaining hemostasis.

Thrombomodulin is expressed by the endothelial cells together with EPCR to convert protein C into its active form. The activation of protein C triggers the inactivation of factor Va and factor VIIIa, causing a block in thrombin production.[8] Calcium and protein S, a glycoprotein made in the endothelium, act as cofactors with protein C to inactivate factor Va. Protein S is also vitamin K dependent.[9]

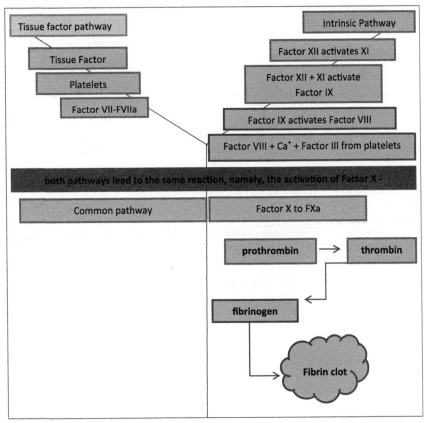

Fig. 3. The clotting cascade. (*Data from* Refs.[3–6])

PLATELETS

Platelets are small, irregularly shaped cell fragments, with an average life span of 5 to 9 days. The normal platelet count ranges from 150,000 to 400,000 platelets per μL in a healthy individual. Platelets play a major role in the formation of the primary hemostatic plug when the vessel wall is injured. Platelets accompanied by von Willebrand factor (vWF) interact and adhere to the site of the injury in the vessel wall as previously discussed. The severity of thrombocytopenia is graded (**Table 1**) and bleeding time is not

Table 1 Grades of thrombocytopenia	
Grades of Thrombocytopenia	**Platelet Counts**
Grade 1	75,000 to 150,000/μL
Grade 2	50,000 to 75,000/μL
Grade 3	25,000 to 50,000/μL
Grade 4	Below 25,000/μL

Data from Sekhon SS, Roy V. Thrombocytopenia in adults: a practical approach to evaluation and management. South Med J 2006;99(5):491–8.

usually prolonged until the platelet count is below 100,000/μL. As long as platelet counts are above 20,000/μL, clinical manifestations are generally mild.[9]

Mild to moderate thrombocytopenia (grade 2–3) is noted in up to 30% of patients with CLD,[3,10] with higher rates noted in patients with end-stage liver disease. Appropriate platelet counts for invasive procedures such as a liver transplant or liver biopsy varies considerably from practice to practice. The American Association for the Study of Liver Diseases (AASLD) position paper[11] specifies standard percutaneous liver biopsy is often withheld in patients with a PT-INR above 1.5. However, it is critical to emphasize that the relationship of coagulation profiles to the risk of bleeding in patients with chronic, as well as acute, liver disease is uncertain.[11] The AASLD also stipulates the decision to perform liver biopsy or invasive procedures in the presence of abnormal laboratory is a decision for the practitioner.[11,12] Therefore, patients should be evaluated on an individual basis and the risks and benefits examined. There is no specific PT-INR and/or platelet count cutoff at or above which potentially adverse bleeding can be reliably predicted.[11] However, a platelet count of 50×10^9 per liter or 50,000 is acceptable in most situations.[12] Bleeding time, an indirect measure of platelet function, is prolonged in up to 40% of patients with cirrhosis.[10]

FIBRINOLYSIS

Fibrinolysis is the process through which fibrin clots are dissolved by the action of plasmin.[12,13] In fibrinolysis, a proenzyme plasminogen is converted into plasmin that breaks down fibrin. The conversion is tightly controlled by antifibrinolytic proteins such as plasminogen activator inhibitor type 1 (PAI-1), plasmin inhibitors (mainly alpha1-plasmin inhibitor), and thrombin-activatable fibrinolysis inhibitor (TAFI).[13,14] These antifibrinolytics are synthesized by the liver, with the exception of tissue plasminogen activator (tPA), which is produced by endothelial cells.[14] The balance between fibrinolysis and antifibrinolysis is important to prevent unwanted plasmin generation as well as hyperfibrinolysis or hypofibrinolysis.[15] The possibility of hyperfibrinolysis in patients with liver disease being linked to TAFI is currently under investigation.[15] In hepatic dysfunction, plasminogen and tPA levels are increased.[15] Furthermore, PAI-1, which hinders tPA, is also increased.[16] Fibrin levels are often normal in stable liver disease but decrease as liver disease progresses. The balance between profibrinolytic and antifibrinolytic pathways is in a state of instability in liver dysfunction. Further instability occurs in the presence of infection or thrombocytopenia.[17]

PT AND INR

PT and INR are frequently used to assess coagulopathy (**Fig. 4**). The PT is a good predictor of liver damage. However, evidence suggests that the PT-INR as an indicator of coagulopathy in liver disease may be misleading.[16] The PT evaluates the extrinsic pathway and measures vitamin K-dependent factors. PT is only affected by five clotting factors (eg, factors VII, X, V, II, and fibrinogen). The maintenance of homeostasis requires a balance between procoagulants and anticoagulants. The plasma and reagents used to perform the PT-INR tests does not contain thrombomodulin, a transmembrane protein in the vascular endothelial cells, which activates protein C. The PT-INR test only measures thrombin generated in plasma as a function of procoagulants. The thrombin inhibited by anticoagulants, such as protein C, is not incorporated in the PT-INR test. Therefore, the test's ability to assess the risk of hemorrhage in liver disease is questionable.[14]

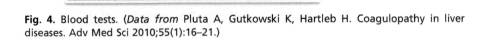

Blood Test

Prothrombin Time (PT) and International Normalized Ratio

- Evaluates Factor VII, FX, FII and Fibrinogen
- Only measures thrombin generated in plasma, but not thrombin inhibited by protein C.
- Prolonged in liver disease
- To monitor Coumadin

Partial Prothrombin (PTT) or Activated Partial Thromboplastin Time (aPTT)

- Evaluated Coagulation Factor XII, XI, IX, VII, X, II (prothrombin), and I (Fibrinogen)
- To monitor standard (unfractionated, UF) heparin anticoagulation therapy
- Normal to slightly prolonged in liver disease

D-Dimer

- Evaluates the acutal time it takes the blood to clot

Fibrinogen level

- Measures the quality of the fibrinogen
- Used after bleeding and transfusion therapy

Fig. 4. Blood tests. (*Data from* Pluta A, Gutkowski K, Hartleb H. Coagulopathy in liver diseases. Adv Med Sci 2010;55(1):16–21.)

PARTIAL PT OR ACTIVATED PARTIAL THROMBOPLASTIN TIME

The partial PT (PTT) measures the intrinsic and common coagulation pathways. The PTT evaluates the coagulation factors XII, XI, IX, VIII, X, V, II (prothrombin), and I (fibrinogen). Activated partial thromboplastin time (aPTT) has been widely used during the last 10 years, but fails to be an accurate predictor of thrombotic or bleeding risks because it only evaluates the coagulation factors VII, X, V, II, and I (fibrinogen) and is often elevated in patients with liver disease. The PTT is prolonged in patients with factor deficiencies in severe liver disease. Because aPTT only addresses the procoagulants, and not the anticoagulants, the effectiveness in predicting a bleeding event or coagulation imbalance in patients with liver disease has been called into question.[17]

Thromboelastograms (TEGs) are being used more frequently to predict bleeding in patients undergoing cardiac surgery and in critically ill patients.[10] The TEG study analyzes whole blood coagulation by including the effects of red blood cells and platelets, along with the clotting factors. Such analysis is more complete and descriptive than the PT and aPTT.[12]

ACUTE LIVER FAILURE

Management of acute liver failure (ALF) requires a multisystem approach. Often, this disease process is accompanied by hepatic encephalopathy, the potential for cerebral edema, renal failure, and hypoxia from impaired oxygen exchange, as well as cardiovascular involvement.[8] ALF is commonly described as the development of coagulopathy, usually with an INR of greater than 1.5, and any degree of mental alteration (encephalopathy) in a patient without preexisting cirrhosis and with an illness of less than 26 weeks duration.[2,18] A hallmark of ALF is depressed synthesis of most procoagulants. The most common procoagulants affected are factors II, V, VII, and X. Spontaneous and iatrogenic bleeding after invasive procedures are two major concerns when coagulation is altered.[2]

Evidence indicates that prolonged INR values (INR 1.5–5.0 in the absence of anticoagulants), typically observed in approximately 80% of ALF patients, are often misleading as an indicator of the severity of coagulopathy in liver failure. However, an elevated INR is part of the accepted definition of liver disease, unless accompanied by complications of coexisting portal hypertension, sepsis, and/or renal failure.[2,16,19] Bleeding in patients with ALF is generally occult bleeding, consistent with oozing from mucosal lesion most often found as superficial gastric erosion, and is generally treated with histamine 2 receptor antagonist or proton pump inhibitors.[2]

ORTHOTROPIC LIVER TRANSPLANT

Orthotropic liver transplant (OLT) is the only effective therapy for patients with ALF who fail to recover spontaneously and constitutes 6% of all liver transplants in the United States.[18] The American Liver Foundation currently estimates more than 6000 transplants are done annually.[19,20] The risks of bleeding and transfusion in OLT are determined by the patient's age, severity of liver disease, and preoperative hemoglobin and plasma fibrinogen values.[21] The incidence of perioperative bleeding has also decreased during the last 10 years and the need for blood transfusions has decreased by 55%.[22] The decreased need for transfusions is likely due to improved techniques and better management of patients to reduce blood loss, such as antifibrinolytic drugs and fluid restriction.[21,22] Centers are now reporting liver transplantation without any need for blood transfusion in up to 30% of patients[21,23] (see later discussion).

CHRONIC LIVER FAILURE

CLD, such as cirrhosis, is associated with an alteration in primary and secondary hemostasis resulting from decreased production of liver proteins. The result is increased bleeding episodes. The causes may include a wide range of conditions from viral (cytomegalovirus, Epstein-Barr, and hepatitis A or B) to toxicity from medications.[9] CLD also results from alcohol abuse and conditions such as NAFLD, right-sided heart failure, and autoimmune disease.[6,9,24]

The hemostatic abnormality seen in patients with CLD seems to be an attempt to rebalance hemostasis. Thrombocytopenia, which is commonly seen in CLD, would normally impair hemostasis. However, the decreased number and function of the platelets are accompanied by an increase in levels of vWF, which promotes hemostasis and attempts to compensate partially for change in clotting ability produced by thrombocytopenia. Furthermore, low levels of factors II, V, VIII, IX, X, and Xa, which act as procoagulants, are accompanied by decreased levels of natural anticoagulants such as protein C, protein S, and antithrombin. The body's attempt to return to a state of balance is not as stable as the hemostatic balance in healthy individuals.[16] This rebalanced system is more vulnerable compared with healthy individuals and, therefore, it can more easily change to either a hypocoagulable or hypercoagulable state.[24]

CIRRHOSIS

Liver cirrhosis is a chronic degenerative condition. Bleeding diathesis associated with esophageal varices is the most common bleeding event seen with cirrhosis.[25] However, in cirrhosis the bleeding results from vascular abnormities and portal hypertension, which creates an increase in vascular pressure.[25] Therefore, the bleeding event is more mechanical in nature than the result of coagulopathy. A history of bleeding, presence and size of esophageal varices, degree of portal hypertension, and presence of comorbid conditions (eg, renal failure or anemia) represents a better predictive value of bleeding in cirrhotic patients than routine coagulation tests.[13]

HYPERCOAGULABILITY

Patients with hepatic coagulopathy were thought to be "auto-anticoagulated" because of the prolonged PT.[26] Studies have shown that 0.5% to 1.9% of patients with liver disease develop deep vein thrombosis or pulmonary emboli. Although bleeding is the most common concern for patients with liver disease, hypercoagulability can create life-threatening complications. The most significant complications are portal vein thrombosis (PVT), clotting of extracorporeal circulation devices, and thrombotic occlusion of intrahepatic blood vessels further damaging the liver.[27]

In a study of subjects with liver failure, the presence of PVT was reported to be as high as 26.72% in those with cirrhosis.[15] Coagulation-related PLT, PT, aPTT, fibrinogen levels, and anticoagulation factor antithrombin-III displayed significant correlations with liver dysfunction, but did not correlate with the formation of PVT.[28] PVT is a cause of portal hypertension and develops in 5% to 20% of patients with cirrhosis.[28] Early recognition and treatment of PVT may prevent gastrointestinal hemorrhage in cirrhotic patients. Zhang and colleagues[28] identified a correlation between protein C and protein S, both were inversely correlated with PVT. Protein C is a major physiologic anticoagulant and is enhanced by protein S.[28] PVT can be diagnosed by Doppler ultrasonography, CT scan, or MRI.[28]

Disseminated intravascular coagulation (DIC) has also been reported in patients with cirrhosis. DIC is a process of both clot formation and clot lysis. It is characterized by elevated PT, aPTT, thrombocytopenia, and fibrin products, as well as elevated d-dimer, fragments of previous fibrin modulators.[26]

EVIDENCED-BASED CARE

Detecting bleeding diathesis involves vigilance and close observation. Frequently observed are positive guaiac stools, the presence of hematuria, and changes in skin integrity in the form of petechiae, ecchymosis, and hematomas. More subtle signs of bleeding include changes in level of consciousness, restlessness, anxiety, unstable blood pressure, and increased abdominal girth.[29] Blood transfusions can be complicated and lead to cardiovascular overload, acute lung injury, noncardiogenic pulmonary edema, and possible transfusion reactions.[30] Patients receiving blood transfusions must be monitored for respiratory distress, pulmonary congestion, and decreased oxygenation.[29] Achieving a balance between the patient's needs and transfusions is important in the management of patients with liver disease. The goal is to maintain hemoglobin (Hgb) around 8 g/dL not to exceed 9 g/dL.[23,24,30] Transfusions are generally not initiated until the Hgb drops to 7.5 or lower. In particular, there are little published data in support of red blood cell transfusion when the Hgb level is more than 7 g/dL.[21,22,29] The clinical practice guidelines from the American Association of Blood Banks[30] recommends adhering to a restrictive transfusion strategy (7–8 g/dL) in hospitalized, stable patients; suggests adhering to a restrictive strategy in hospitalized patients with preexisting cardiovascular disease; and considering transfusion for symptomatic patients or a hemoglobin level of 8 g/dL or less.[30] Patients with bleeding should be investigated for superimposed causes of coagulopathy such as infections and renal failure.

Platelet transfusions in patients with CLD may be considered if the platelet count is less than 50,000/mm. Target platelet counts to be achieved in CLD patients are more than 70,000/mm.[31] Vitamin K, although slow to respond, is frequently prescribed in the management of patients with end-stage liver disease who demonstrate abnormalities in their coagulation parameters (INR greater than 5.0). Vitamin K does return the PT-INR to normal; however, given the only improvement is related to the PT and PTT, there is some question as to its usefulness.[32] Recombinant factor VIIa concentrate in low doses (80 µg–1.2 µg) may be considered and has been shown to stop bleeding. However, recombinant factor VIIa improves PT and clot formation without affecting fibrinolysis[31] and, as a result, the use of it in the management of overt bleeding from OLT is still being debated.[33] Platelets are considered if the platelet count is less than 50,000/mm.[30] Fresh frozen plasma (FFP) is usually used in the bleeding patient and contains all coagulation factors, inhibitors of coagulation, and fibrinolytic factors. FFP is also helpful as a volume expander (**Fig. 5**).[31] FFP has unpredictable response in decompensated liver cirrhosis and is associated with increased side effects, such as exacerbation of portal hypertension and risk of infection.[31] Desmopressin and prothrombin complex concentrate are available, as well as cryoprecipitate and recombinant factor VIIa. The effect is immediate and transient. Repeated dosing is required and is very costly; however, it should be considered for patients with bleeding that is not responsive to intravenous fluids and blood transfusions.[32]

A medication review is also required in the presence of thrombocytopenia to rule out a drug-induced cause. Thrombocytopenia is a common side effect of many drugs, particularly chemotherapy drugs and valproic acid. Several other medications are

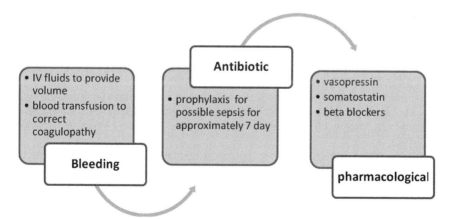

Fig. 5. Managing bleeding events. (*Data from* Refs.[9,18,29,31])

also associated with thrombocytopenia, such as furosemide (Lasix), nonsteroidal anti-inflammatory drugs, penicillin, quinidine, quinine, ranitidine, amiodarone, digoxin, fluconazole, heparin, and sulfonamides.[9] Providers should discontinue use of platelet inhibitors and replace heparin line flushes with saline. Evidence of heparin-induced complications supports the use of nonheparinized saline flushing protocols. Heparin-induced thrombocytopenia can develop with minimal heparin doses such as those used to flush.[34] Finally, transfusions may be necessary to maintain a balance between procoagulant and anticoagulant factors; however, the potential risks and benefits of transfusing need to be examined.

SUMMARY

Coagulation abnormalities and bleeding diathesis are frequently a concern in patients with chronic and acute liver disease.[35–37] Hemostasis imbalance and rebalance contributes to a risk of bleeding in the patients with liver disease.[14,25,36] Improved techniques and therapies to improve hemostasis have resulted in a decrease in bleeding severity and a reduction in blood transfusions.

The current PT and aPTT laboratory tests fail to detect the hemostasis rebalance related bleeding tendencies and do not accurately predict bleeding events in patients with liver disease. The use of thrombin generation assays (TGA), currently being reviewed, may be a more useful method of assessing bleeding potential or hemostasis imbalances. Because many functions of thrombin regulate or directly cause clot formation, thrombin generation is considered a good marker of global hemostasis.[37]

Further studies into the use of TEG for projecting bleeding events in patients with liver failure may be beneficial.[15] Continued research is needed in both the prediction of bleeding events (ie, TGA and TEG) and the management of the bleeding events in patients with liver failure. As new evidence is introduced, the original impression of bleeding tendencies may not be correct. The bleeding diathesis seems to be the result of dysfunction in coagulation, anticoagulation, and fibrinolytic systems, instead of just a single system.[17,28] Transfusion practices should be evaluated to minimize the related complications.

REFERENCES

1. Younossi ZM, Stepanova M, Afendy M, et al. Changes in the prevalence of the most common causes of chronic liver diseases in the United States from 1988 to 2008. Clin Gastroenterol Hepatol 2011;9(6):524–30.e1.
2. Munoz SJ, Stravitz RT, Gabriel DA. Coagulopathy of acute liver failure. Clin Liver Dis 2009;13(1):95–107.
3. Caldwell SH, Sanyal AJ. Coagulation disorders and bleeding in liver disease: future directions. Clin Liver Dis 2009;13(1):155–7.
4. Lisman T, Leebeek FW. Hemostatic alterations in liver disease: a review on pathophysiology, clinical consequences, and treatment. Dig Surg 2007;24(4):250–8.
5. Mertens K, Meijer AB. Factors VIII and V swap fatty feet. Blood 2012;120(9): 1761–3.
6. Monroe DM, Hoffman M. The coagulation cascade in cirrhosis. Clin Liver Dis 2009;13(1):1–9.
7. Esmon CT. The protein C pathway. Chest 2003;124(Suppl 3):26S–32S.
8. D'Alessio S, Genua M, Vetrano S. The protein C pathway in intestinal barrier function: challenging the hemostasis paradigm. Ann N Y Acad Sci 2012;1258(1): 78–85.

9. Sekhon SR, Roy V. Thrombocytopenia in adults: a practical approach to evaluation and management. South Med J 2006;99(5):491–8.
10. Thachil J. Relevance of clotting tests in liver disease. Postgrad Med J 2008; 84(990):177–81.
11. Rockey DC, Caldwell SH, Goodman ZD, et al, American Association for the Study of Liver Diseases. Liver biopsy. Hepatology 2009;49(3):1011–44.
12. Pluta A, Gutkowski K, Hartleb H. Coagulopathy in liver diseases. Adv Med Sci 2010;55(1):16–21.
13. Hoekstra J, Guimarães AH, Leebeek FW, et al. Impaired fibrinolysis as a risk factor for Budd-Chiari syndrome. Blood 2010;115(2):388–95.
14. Tripodi A, Mannucci PM. The coagulopathy of chronic liver disease. N Engl J Med 2011;365(2):147–56.
15. Hodge A, Crispin P. Coagulopathy in liver disease: the whole is greater than the sum of its parts. J Gastroenterol Hepatol 2010;25:1–2.
16. Agarwal B, Wright G, Gatt A, et al. Evaluation of coagulation abnormalities in acute liver failure. J Hepatol 2012;57:780–6.
17. Warnaar N, Lisman T, Porte RJ. The two tales of coagulation in liver transplatation. Curr Opin Organ Transplant 2008;13:298–303.
18. Sargent S. An overview of acute liver failure: managing rapid deterioration. Gastrointest Nurs 2010;8(9):36–42.
19. Tripodi A. Tests of coagulation in liver disease. Clin Liver Dis 2009;13(1):55–61.
20. American Liver Foundation. Liver transplants. 2013. Available at: http://www.liverfoundation.org/abouttheliver/info/transplant/. Accessed August 12, 2013.
21. Sabate A, Dalmau A, Koo M, et al. Coagulopathy management in liver transplantation. Transplant Proc 2012;44(6):1523–5.
22. Feltracco P, Brezzi M, Barbieri S, et al. Blood loss, predictors of bleeding, transfusion practice and strategies of blood cell salvaging during liver transplantation. World J Hepatol 2013;5(1):1–15.
23. De Boer MT, Christensen MC, Asmussen M, et al. The impact of intraoperative transfusion of platelets and red blood cells on survival after liver transplantation. Anesth Analg 2008;106(1):32–44.
24. Van Der Werf J, Porte RJ, Lisman T. Hemostasis in patients with liver disease. Acta Gastroenterol Belg 2009;72(4):433–40.
25. Lisman T, Porte RJ. Rebalanced hemostasis in patients with liver disease: evidence and clinical consequences. Blood 2010;116(6):878–85.
26. Van Theil DH, George M, Mindikoglu AL, et al. Coagulation and fibrinolysis in individuals with advanced liver disease. Turk J Gastroenterol 2004;15(2):67–72.
27. Ng VL. Liver disease, coagulation testing, and hemostasis. Clin Lab Med 2009; 29(2):265–82.
28. Zhang D, Hao J, Yang N. Protein C and D-dimer are related to portal vein thrombosis in patients with liver cirrhosis. J Gastroenterol Hepatol 2010;25(1):116–21.
29. Dressler DK. Coagulopathy in the intensive care unit. Crit Care Nurse 2012;32(5): 48–60.
30. Carson JL, Grossman BJ, Kleinman S, et al. Red blood cell transfusion: a clinical practice guideline from the AABB*. Ann Intern Med 2012;157(1):49–58.
31. Amarapurkar PD, Amarapurkar DN. Management of coagulopathy in patients with decompensated liver cirrhosis. Int J Hepatol 2011;2011:695470.
32. Saja MF, Abdo AA, Sanai FM, et al. The coagulopathy of liver disease: does vitamin K help. Blood Coagul Fibrinolysis 2013;24(1):10–7.
33. Mayer SA, Brun NC, Begtrup K, et al. Efficacy and safety of recombinant activated factor VII for acute intracerebral hemorrhage. N Engl J Med 2008;358(20):2127–37.

34. Mathers D. Evidence-based practice: improving outcomes for patients with a central venous access device. J Vasc Access 2011;16(2):64–72.
35. Lisman T, Caldwell SH, Burroughs AK, et al. Hemostasis and thrombosis in patients with liver disease: the ups and downs. J Hepatol 2010;53(2):362–71.
36. Tripodi A, Primignani M, Chantarangkul V, et al. The coagulopathy of cirrhosis assessed by thromboelastometry and its correlation with conventional coagulation parameters. Thromb Res 2009;124(1):132–6.
37. Tripodi A, Anstee QM, Sogaard KK, et al. Hypercoagulability in cirrhosis: causes and consequences. J Thromb Haemost 2011;9(9):1713–23.

Critical Care Issues in Management of High-Grade Lymphoma

Jennifer K. Johnson, MSN, RN, ACNS-BC, AOCNS[a,*],
Elizabeth Sorensen, MSN, RN, ACNS-BC, AOCNS[b]

KEYWORDS

- Burkitt lymphoma • Renal failure • HIV • AIDS • Tumor lysis syndrome
- Inferior vena cava obstruction

KEY POINTS

- Lymphoma is a heterogeneous malignancy of the lymphatic system with presentations ranging from insidious to fulminant.
- Although very aggressive, BL can be highly treatable.
- Patients with BL often present with conditions that warrant critical care.
- TLS is a phenomenon seen in rapidly proliferating malignancies, usually in response to rapid cell death in response to cytotoxic therapies.
- Follicular lymphoma is unique because it has the potential to transform into the more aggressive DLBCL, with an estimated risk at 3% per year after initial diagnosis.
- Transformed DLBCL have poorer outcomes compared with de novo (newly diagnosed) DLBCL and therefore accurate diagnosis with prompt treatment is critical.

INTRODUCTION

Lymphoma is a heterogeneous malignancy of the lymphatic system with presentations ranging from insidious to fulminant. Based on the 2008 World Health Organization classification, there are close to 70 subtypes of lymphoma, generally divided into Hodgkin and non-Hodgkin lymphoma (NHL), both of which are further subdivided based on clinical and pathologic behavior.[1] Lymphoma is not rare; NHL is the fifth most common malignancy in the United Kingdom. In the United States, NHL

Disclosures: None.
[a] Nocturnal Program, MD Anderson Cancer Center, The University of Texas, 1515 Holcombe Boulevard, Unit 0379, Houston, TX 77030, USA; [b] Lymphoma and Myeloma Department, MD Anderson Cancer Center, The University of Texas, 1515 Holcombe Boulevard, Unit 429, Houston, TX 77030, USA
* Corresponding author.
E-mail address: jkjohnson@mdanderson.org

accounted for more than 65,000 new cases in 2007 and more than 20,000 deaths in 2008.[2] This article compares the presentation of two patients who were seen in the emergency department (ED) on the same day at our institution (a National Comprehensive Cancer Network site) with life-threatening complications arising from high-grade lymphomas of very different origin, highlighting the varied presentations of high-grade lymphoma. Additionally, the cause, evaluation, and management of critical care issues in aggressive lymphoma are described.

CASE PRESENTATION #1
Burkitt Lymphoma

The first patient is Mr A, a 42-year-old Hispanic man who presented with a massive right axillary mass and abdominal pain. His medical history is significant for hypertension, non–insulin dependent diabetes, and morbid obesity. He denies known history of renal failure. For 10 days before his presentation at our ED, the patient had noticed a rapidly enlarging, painless mass in his right axilla. Over the last 4 days, the patient has complained of anorexia, early satiety, and progressive right upper quadrant pain for which he has been taking 12 to 16 ibuprofen tablets daily without relief.

Eventually, the pain led the patient to present to a community ED, where he underwent computed tomography (CT) of the chest, abdomen, and pelvis and was informed that he had widespread metastatic disease of unknown type. Mr A was advised to seek treatment from an oncologist and self-referred to our institution. On further questioning in our ED, the patient endorses increasing abdominal girth, malaise, and multiple episodes of drenching night sweats over the last 2 weeks. He denies other constitutional symptoms including weight loss, cough, dyspnea, nausea, vomiting, or diarrhea. The patient denied a history of sick contacts, foreign travel, history of intravenous drug abuse, tobacco, or alcohol abuse beyond one to two drinks weekly. The patient states he is in a long-term monogamous heterosexual relationship, has no tattoos, and has never had sex with another male.

The combination of localized painless lymphadenopathy, drenching night sweats, and abdominal symptoms raises concern for development of lymphoma. Coupled with the sudden onset and rapid progression of symptoms, the patient's presentation suggests a very aggressive disease. Clinical presentation led to high suspicion of aggressive lymphoma, such as Burkitt lymphoma (BL). Mr A urgently underwent a fine-needle aspiration of the axillary mass, which revealed BL, BCL-6$^+$, CD19$^+$, CD20$^+$, CD22$^+$, FMC7$^+$, and kappa light chain–positive, BCL-2, and Epstein-Barr virus negative. Ki-67, a measure of cell proliferation, is 100%.

BL is a rare, highly aggressive mature B-cell lymphoma accounting for less than 1% of all NHL.[3] BL is considered the "fastest growing human tumor," and is invariably fatal without treatment.[4] Survival is reckoned in weeks to months without therapy.[4] Symptoms are related to rapid turnover of mature B lymphocytes, extent of extranodal involvement, or invasion into organs. BL has three variants: (1) endemic, (2) sporadic, and (3) immunodeficiency related.[5] Endemic BL, a childhood disease, is usually found in equatorial Africa and presents as painless neck, jaw, or facial masses.[5] Abdominal, gonadal, and skeletal presentations are also seen. Sporadic forms of BL generally present with bone marrow involvement and abdominal disease, with diagnosis often precipitated by bowel obstruction or intussusception caused by mass effect. Other presentations include intracardiac disease, pancreatitis, ovarian or breast involvement, and occasional skin lesions. Generalized lymphadenopathy is less common.[5] Finally, immunodeficiency-related BL usually presents with localized lymphadenopathy and usually spares the bone marrow.[5] Whether innate or acquired, immune deficiency is commonly associated with malignancy in general, and lymphoma and leukemia specifically.[3]

Infectious disease accounts for approximately 25% of worldwide malignancies. Generally, there is a long latent period between infection and manifestation of malignancies, and only a small percentage of those infected eventually develop malignancies.[6] However, latent EBV is almost invariably associated with endemic BL and occasionally with sporadic BL.[6] Other infectious diseases strongly associated with lymphoma include *Helicobacter pylori*, human herpesvirus 8, human T-lymphotrophic virus, hepatitis C virus, and EBV.

In the immune-deficient subtype, latent EBV is most commonly seen in the HIV-positive patient, where the virus is actually seen inside the malignant cells.[3] Immune-deficient BL is also strongly associated with HIV infection and constitutes an AIDS-defining illness.[7] Fortunately, in the age of highly active antiretroviral therapy (HAART), survival of HIV-associated BL closely mirrors that of non–HIV associated BL.[8]

Although very aggressive, BL can be highly treatable. Overall survival for adult patients younger than age 60 approaches 90%.[4] The survival rate is predicated on prompt diagnosis of the disease state. Rapidly enlarging lymphadenopathy with fulminant symptoms should always raise suspicion for development of a high-grade lymphoma. High-grade lymphomas, including BL, require urgent evaluation and treatment and should be treated as medical emergencies.[2] Physical examination findings are dictated by disease site. Abdominal involvement is common in nonendemic BL, reported as between 60% and 90% of cases, depending on source. Clinical signs range from abdominal tenderness, hepatosplenomegaly, or ascites to frank peritonitis in the case of perforation. Approximately 25% of all BL have ileocecal involvement.[4] The next most common site of involvement is head/neck, including cervical and supraclavicular lymph nodes, sinuses, or tonsils.[4] Central nervous system (CNS) involvement is relatively rare, except in cases of HIV-associated BL, and varies from cranial nerve deficits, headache, paraplegia, or other symptoms suggestive of spinal cord involvement to meningeal signs, visual disturbances, or vague, nonspecific neurologic symptoms. Cranial nerve involvement most commonly manifests as cranial nerve III and/or VII deficits. Patients may report early satiety, nausea and vomiting, fatigue, unexplained fevers, gastrointestinal bleeding, or soaking night sweats.[5]

The rapid progression of BL necessitates an urgent diagnostic evaluation. Diagnostic work-up includes obtaining adequate tissue specimen to obtain at least one paraffin block representative of tumor and flow cytometry and molecular genetic analysis. If specimens are nondiagnostic, they should not be interpreted as negative. Rebiopsy is essential.[9] Baseline evaluation of BL is shown in **Box 1**.

Critical Illness Associated with BL

Patients with BL often present with conditions that warrant critical care. Mr A presented with acute kidney injury requiring renal-replacement therapy and tumor lysis syndrome (TLS). The presence of acute kidney injury in newly diagnosed hematologic malignancies is associated with lower rates of remission and with increased mortality.[10] The poor prognosis is caused by several factors, including the disease itself and treatment-related toxicities.[10] Disease-related factors include obstructive uropathies caused by mass effect, renal infiltration with disease, or TLS, in addition to sepsis or hypoperfusion. Treatment-related toxicities include treatment with nephrotoxic chemotherapies and antibiotics. Impaired renal function can lead to incorrect chemotherapy dosing with underdosing leading to increased incidence of treatment failure, and overdosing to increased renal toxicity. Worsening increased short-term toxicity and lower response rates have been correlated with severity of kidney injury.[10]

> **Box 1**
> **Baseline evaluation for suspected Burkitt lymphoma**
>
> - Excisional biopsy or core needle biopsy is strongly recommended; fine-needle aspiration is generally inadequate. If specimen is nondiagnostic, rebiopsy is essential
> - CT of neck, chest, abdomen, and pelvis with triple contrast
> - Positron emission tomography/CT scan
> - Chest radiograph, posteroanterior and lateral
> - Echocardiogram
> - Bilateral bone marrow biopsy and aspiration
> - Lumbar puncture with cytology evaluation
> - Complete blood count with differential, electrolytes, total bilirubin, aspartate aminotransferase, alanine aminotransferase, alkaline phosphatase, albumin, serum calcium, uric acid, phosphorous, magnesium, blood urea nitrogen, creatinine (Cr), and lactate dehydrogenase
> - HIV 1 and 2 and hepatitis B and C serology
> - All women of child-bearing potential must have a pregnancy test
> - Physical examination findings and Eastern Cooperative Oncology Group or Karnofsky performance status should be accurately evaluated and documented
> - Magnetic resonance imaging with gadolinium contrast of brain (preferred) or CT brain with contrast of any patient with CNS symptoms
> - Select cases may require upper and/or lower endoscopy to evaluate gastrointestinal symptoms
> - Potential loss of fertility should be discussed

TLS is a phenomenon seen in rapidly proliferating malignancies, usually in response to rapid cell death in response to cytotoxic therapies. Spontaneous tumor lysis also occurs. The syndrome manifests as a wide range of metabolic derangements resulting from "rapid release of intracellular metabolites such as nucleic acids, proteins, phosphorous, and potassium from lysed cells" resulting in elevations in uric acid, phosphorous, and potassium, and possible hypocalcemia.[11] These abnormalities overwhelm the body's compensatory mechanisms, resulting in renal failure, arrhythmias, cardiac arrest, seizures, and death.[12] Risk for tumor lysis is stratified by disease type and disease burden, elevations in WBC and lactate dehydrogenase (LDH), and presence of pre-existing kidney disease. BL is considered high-risk for development of TLS.

All patients with newly diagnosed BL should be treated with rasburicase, aggressive hydration, and serial measurement of electrolytes, with correction of hyperkalemia, hyperphosphatemia, and hypocalcemia.[11] Rasburicase, approved by the Food and Drug Administration for treatment and prophylaxis of TLS in 2002, catalyzes the enzymatic oxidation of relatively insoluble uric acid to allantoin, a more soluble metabolite. This results in reduced uric acid levels. The presence of a G6PD deficiency is an absolute contraindication to the administration of rasburicase because it leads to methemoglobinemia. Because screening for G6PD deficiencies is not readily available in medical emergencies, patients of African-American or Mediterranean descent should be closely evaluated for possible G6PD deficiency.[13] If rasburicase is contraindicated, allopurinol may be used. Renal-replacement therapy should be considered for recalcitrant electrolyte abnormalities, severe acid-base imbalance, or oliguria leading to volume overload.[11]

Successful treatment of Mr A's disease has several complicating factors. First, he has pre-existing renal failure on initial evaluation, and laboratory data suggestive of spontaneous TLS (**Table 1**). Mr A's previous history of type II diabetes and uncontrolled hypertension, and recent nonsteroidal anti-inflammatory drug abuse, makes evaluation of his baseline renal function difficult. On initial imaging, Mr A was found to have extensive lymphomatous infiltration in both kidneys, which further compromises renal function. He was eventually given a dose of rasburicase and started on renal-replacement therapy for correction of electrolytes and acid-base balance. Mr A was able to start his first cycle of chemotherapy within 24 hours of his initial presentation to the ED and was eventually able to be discharged from the hospital.

Baseline evaluation also revealed a new diagnosis of HIV and evidence of previous cytomegalovirus exposure. Mr A was started on HAART therapy, which put him at increased risk of developing immune reconstitution inflammatory syndrome in which previously unknown infections are unmasked as immune system recovery develops.[6] Outcomes for patients with AIDS-related lymphomas, when treated with appropriate HAART and chemotherapy, are very similar to those without AIDS, although there is increased risk of infectious disease and immune reconstitution inflammatory syndrome–related complications.[14] He has been hospitalized several times since initial evaluation for findings of parainfluenza type 3 pneumonia and exacerbations of chronic kidney disease. After two cycles of chemotherapy, repeat imaging showed no active tumor, and the patient was fortunately found to be in complete metabolic response. Because of the excellent response to treatment, the patient will receive an additional four cycles of chemotherapy.

Although BL is known to represent a highly aggressive lymphoma, indolent lymphomas can also exhibit aggressive behaviors. Slow-growing lymphomas, such as follicular lymphoma, are rarely considered curable, although achieving remission that results in a waxing and waning course is common.[15] However, a relatively small

Table 1 Significant abnormal laboratory data		
Laboratory	Value	Reference Range
Na	130	135–147 mEq/L
BUN	38	8–20 mg/dL
Cr	3.9	0.7–1.3 mg/dL
Alb	2.7	3.5–4.7 g/dL
AST	91	15–46 IU/L
ALT	25	7–56 IU/L
Uric acid	11.5	2.6–7.1 mg/dL
Phos	5.3	2.5–4.5 mg/dL
Lipase	431	23–300 IU/L
Amylase	53	30–110 IU/L
LDH	2985	313–618 IU/L
HCT	31.5	40%–54%
Hgb	11.1	14–18 g/dL

Abbreviations: Alb, albumin; ALT, alanine aminotransferase; AST, aspartate aminotransferase; BUN, blood urea nitrogen; Cr, creatinine; HCT, hematocrit.

Adapted from The International Non-Hodgkin's Lymphoma Prognostic Factors Project. N Engl J Med 1993;329:989; with permission.

number of these lymphomas transform to a more aggressive form. Transformation to a more aggressive form of lymphoma occurs in 25% to 35% of patients over the lifespan of their disease, which often spans decades.[16] In these cases of transformed lymphoma, the malignancy (generally already BCL-2$^+$) acquires an MYC gene rearrangement. The BCL-2 protein is a strongly antiapoptic protein, meaning cells resist programed death, while the MYC gene enhances cell proliferation. Together, these rearrangements result in a rapidly proliferating cell line. Lymphomas with both rearrangements are classified as double-hit lymphomas, and as a result of their mutations, are highly aggressive and highly treatment resistant. Biopsy specimens yielding multiple subtypes of genetically and immunophenotypically distinct forms of lymphoma are occasionally seen. For example, a single biopsy specimen could be comprised of two distinct types of lymphoma (ie, both Hodgkins and follicular). More commonly, a specimen composed of both an indolent and aggressive lymphoma can be expressed, in which a subset of cells have acquired an MYC gene rearrangement. The complex process that leads to this transformation is not yet clearly understood.[15] Our second case presentation highlights the acute presentations often seen with these complex cases.

CASE PRESENTATION #2
Transformed Follicular Lymphoma

Mr B, a 52-year-old man previously treated for stage III, CD10$^+$, CD19$^+$, CD20$^+$, BCL-2$^+$, CD5$^-$ grade 3 follicular lymphoma with R-CHOP (rituxan, cytoxan, adriamycin, and prednisone) for six cycles with complete resolution of lymphadenopathy presents with a 4.3 × 3.2 cm mass in the retroperitoneum. A biopsy shows grade 1 to 2 follicular lymphoma with no evidence of grade 3 component. Follicular lymphoma is classified as grades 1, 2, or 3 based on pattern of aggression, with 3 being the most aggressive. LDH is not elevated. He was observed without therapy for asymptomatic disease. He did not receive any treatment of his lymphoma and resumed his normal activities until 4 months later when he noted a 3-day history of constipation and abdominal pain. The abdominal pain worsened to the point that Mr B became nauseated and could no longer eat. Mr B then presented to his local ED. CT imaging showed a doubling in the size of the retroperitoneal mass over the 4-month period, with interval development of right-sided hydronephrosis and compression of the inferior vena cava caused by mass effect. The mass effect resulted in inferior vena cava syndrome. A biopsy showed BCL2$^+$, CD20$^+$, CD10$^+$ follicular lymphoma with increased large cells and suspicion for aggressive transformation. In this sample, Ki-67 was positive in 40% of all cells. The expression of Ki-67 is associated with cell proliferation and is often correlated with the aggressiveness of the disease.[17] Fluroescence in situ hybridization study showed presence of a clone with MYC gene rearrangement classifying the tumor as double-hit large cell lymphoma. Of note, multiple biopsy specimens were obtained using CT-guided percutaneous core-needle and fine-needle technique for a total of seven specimens to yield sufficient diagnostic material. After a final diagnosis, Mr B presented to discuss chemotherapy and transplant options.

Mr B's case highlights the heterogeneity of lymphoma. The disease varies widely, not only between disease subtypes, but even within a single patient, with a similarly wide range of clinical presentations. NHL or B-cell lymphomas are the most common classification of lymphoma, whereas the aggressive diffuse large B-cell lymphoma (DLBCL) is the most common subtype.[18]

DLBCL is a unique cancer because it is readily curable even when diagnosed at an advanced stage. Approximately 67% of patients are alive and progression-free at

4 years with standard anthracycline and rituximab based therapy.[19] Alternately, DLBCL can be extremely challenging to treat in the relapsed setting, and 10% to 15% exhibit primary refractory disease.[19]

DLBCL accounts for 30% of all newly diagnosed lymphomas and 80% of all aggressive lymphomas, whereas follicular lymphoma is the second most common type of NHL.[14,18] Follicular lymphoma is unique because it has the potential to transform into the more aggressive DLBCL, with an estimated risk at 3% per year after initial diagnosis.[20] Histologic evaluation determines the transformation from indolent to aggressive disease. Factors contributing to increased risk of transformation include high LDH on initial diagnosis; advanced-stage disease (stage III/IV); high International Prognostic Index (IPI) (**Table 2**) or Follicular Lymphoma International Prognostic Index (FLIPI) scores; and grade 3a histology. Both the IPI and FLIPI are models that predict patient outcomes based on clinical characteristics before treatment.[21,22] Transformed DLBCL have poorer outcomes compared with de novo (newly diagnosed) DLBCL and therefore accurate diagnosis with prompt treatment is critical.[23]

Both de novo and transformed DLBCL have similar presentations including B symptoms, fatigue, adenopathy, and occasionally extranodal involvement. B symptoms, which include fever, night sweats, and weight loss, are present in about 30% to 40% of patients with aggressive lymphomas.[24] Fatigue and weakness are also common presenting symptoms with advanced disease or aggressive forms of lymphoma. Most patients present with adenopathy but one-third present with extranodal involvement in sites including gastrointestinal tract, skin, bone marrow, sinuses, genitourinary tract, thyroid, and CNS.[24]

After a person presents with lymphadenopathy or suspicion of lymphoma, obtaining a tissue diagnosis is the next step to effective clinical management. A definitive diagnosis can be made only by excisional or core needle biopsy of involved lymph nodes or tumor tissue.[25] Fine-needle aspiration is often insufficient for diagnosis with many false-negatives.[25] A formal review by a hematopathologist includes morphologic evaluation and immunophenotyping and cytogenetic testing.

Because an aggressive lymphoma can rapidly progress and result in tissue destruction, pain, CNS spread, and acute infection with risk of death, the evaluation process

Table 2
International Prognostic Index

IPI Risk Factors

1. Age >60 y
2. Ann Arbor stage III/IV
3. More than one extranodal site
4. Serum LDH level above normal
5. Eastern Cooperative Oncology Group performance status ≥ 2

Risk Group	IPI Score	Percentage of Patients	5-y Overall Survival	Complete Response Rate
Low	0–1	35%	73%	87%
Low-intermediate	2	27%	51%	67%
High-intermediate	3	22%	43%	55%
High	4–5	16%	26%	44%

The International Prognostic Index (IPI) was specifically designed to predict treatment outcomes and long-term survival in patients with aggressive NHL.

must be expedited. To establish risk stratification and to formulate a treatment plan the initial diagnostic evaluation should include the following[24]:

- Careful history including infectious disease and chemical exposure
- Physical examination with palpation of lymph node stations, liver, spleen, and head-to-toe skin examination
- CT scans of neck, chest, abdomen, and pelvis
- Bilateral bone marrow aspiration and biopsy
- Positron emission tomography/CT scan
- Complete blood count with differential and platelet count
- Upper gastrointestinal endoscopy in patients with gastrointestinal complaints or history of *H pylori*
- Cerebrospinal fluid evaluation and magnetic resonance imaging of brain and spine in patients with CNS complaints or highly aggressive variants

Mr B was initially managed with observation alone because he was asymptomatic and had relatively low-risk disease. His tumor burden, a term that refers to the amount of cancer in the body, was low, his age is younger than 60, and he had no extranodal disease. His IPI score is low, and he had no significant comorbidities. Unfortunately, over a short period of time, the tumor displayed aggressive features including fast growth, and Mr B became symptomatic with profound fatigue, weight loss, and acute pain.

After presenting to the ED with acute abdominal pain, constipation for 3 days, weight loss, and evidence of a large abdominal mass on CT scan, he was admitted directly to the in-patient service with a plan to manage pain, constipation, and nutrition, and to restage his disease, which included rebiopsy of the abdominal mass, positron emission tomography (PET) scan, cerebrospinal fluid analysis, and full laboratory evaluation. His laboratory values were grossly unremarkable with normal LDH and normal blood counts.

PET scan showed a large, dominant hypermetabolic right retroperitoneal mass and infiltrative hypermetabolism in the right renal pelvis and perinephric spaces with maximum standardized uptake value (SUV) of 33.2. Increased fluorodeoxyglucose avidity and higher SUV on PET scans correlate to increased metabolic activity. In the setting of lymphoma, these are markers of more rapidly growing disease. Mr B's values are indicative of very aggressive disease.[26] A core needle biopsy was taken from the mass with the highest SUV on PET. Pathology review and additional genetic testing was performed showing evidence of an MYC gene rearrangement using fluroescence in situ hybridization break apart probe, a technique used to identify chromosomal abnormalities (**Fig. 1**).[27] The combination of the BCL2 translocation and MYC gene rearrangement classifies the tumor as double-hit DLBCL (DH DLBCL). DH DLBCL has been established as a high-risk disease with poorer outcomes with conventional treatments.[28]

After the pathology was confirmed, the patient was started on R-Hyper CVAD (rituximab, hyper Cytoxan, vincristine, doxorubicin, dexamethasone) along with growth factor support. He received two identical cycles of therapy and underwent repeat PET scan before his third planned cycle, which showed dramatic interval metabolic response to therapy with reduction in size and near-complete resolution of fluorodeoxyglucose avidity of the abdominal mass. Because of the aggressive and resistant nature of transformed DLBCL and DH DLBCL, the stem cell transplant (SCT) team was consulted and determined that Mr B was a good candidate for autologous SCT. Patients with transformed DLBCL undergoing autologous SCT have better outcomes than those treated with rituximab-containing regimens alone.[23] Allogeneic SCT is associated with significant treatment-related morbidity and mortality and does not improve outcomes compared with rituximab-containing regimens alone.[23]

A
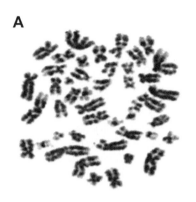

B
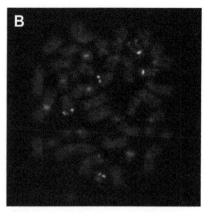

Fig. 1. (*A, B*) Metaphase G-banding and metaphase fluroescence in situ hybridization analysis using LSI IGH/MYC, CEP 8 Tri-color, Dual Fusion Translocation Probe set. (*From* Motlló C, Grau J, Juncá J, et al. Translocation (3;8)(q27;q24) in two cases of triple hit lymphoma. Cancer Genet Cytogenet 2010;203:328–32; with permission.)

SUMMARY

The very different presentations of Mr A and Mr B, seen serially in the ED at our institution, highlight the very heterogeneous presentations of lymphoma. The presenting complaint of both patients was abdominal pain, and both had potential life-threatening conditions necessitating emergent evaluation and treatment in the setting of rapidly progressive disease. Mr A's most urgent issues were acute renal failure and TLS, whereas Mr B was symptomatic and had bulky disease with aggressive transformation. Fortunately, both patients have responded to treatment, and seem to have reasonable chances of long-term survival.

Key diagnostic points in the management of these two cases are suspicion for the presence of a high-grade malignancy, and the need for a sense of urgency in obtaining diagnosis. Because Mr A did not have a diagnosed malignancy, the key laboratory data needed to lead one to the diagnosis of BL was not obtained. The addition of LDH and uric acid to his pending laboratory data and their significantly elevations provided the diagnostic clues for TLS, which in turn led to the initiation of aggressive hydration, rasburicase, and nephrology consult. This initial treatment plan was initiated even before the patient had a firm diagnosis. Mr B was well-known to our institution and was quickly evaluated for disease progression. However, if Mr B, like Mr A, had undergone only a fine-needle aspiration, key pathologic data that showed the transformation to double-hit lymphoma likely would have been missed, leading to possible undertreatment and subsequent treatment failure. Despite lymphoma's many presentations, most remain highly treatable. High-grade disease requires a sense of urgency and appropriate diagnostic evaluation to lead to accurate diagnosis and successful treatment.

REFERENCES

1. Swerdlow S, Campo E, Harris NL, International Agency for Research on Cancer, editors. WHO classification of tumours of haematopoetic and lymphoid tissue. Geneva (Switzerland): World Health Organization; 2008.
2. Shankland KR, Armitage JO, Hancock BW. Non-Hodgkin's lymphoma. Lancet 2012;380:848–57.

3. Wilkins BS. Lymphoma. In: Houston M, Davie B, Harrison R, editors. Blood and bone marrow pathology. 2nd edition. London: Churchill Livingstone; 2011. p. 419–44.

4. Molyneaux EM, Rochford R, Griffin B, et al. Burkitt's lymphoma. Lancet 2012; 379(9822):1234–44. http://dx.doi.org/10.1016/S0140-6736(11)61177-X ISSN: 0140-6736.

5. Kanbar AH, Sacher R, Besa EC, et al. Burkitt and Burkitt's-like lymphoma. 2012. Available at: www.medscape.com. Accessed June 30, 2013.

6. Levine A. Lymphomas and leukemias due to infectious organisms. Hematology 2012;17:87–9. http://dx.doi.org/10.1179/102453312X13336169155934.

7. Fauci AS, Lane HC. Chapter 189. Human immunodeficiency virus disease: AIDS and related disorders. In: Longo DL, Fauci AS, Kasper DL, et al, editors. Harrison's principles of internal medicine. 18th edition. 2012. Available at: http://www.accessmedicine.com/content.aspx?aID=9123335. Accessed April 28, 2013.

8. Petrich AM, Sparano JA, Parech S. Paradigns and contrvoersies in the treatment of HIV-related Burkitt lymphoma. Adv Hematol 2012;2012:403648.

9. Fanale M, Younes A, Reed V, et al. Burkitt's and double-hit lymphoma clinical practice guidelines. 2013. Available at: http://www.mdanderson.org/education-and-research/resources-for-professionals/clinical-tools-and-resources/practice-algorithms/ca-treatment-lymphoma-burkitt-s-web-algorithm.pdf. Accessed April 29, 2013.

10. Canet E, Zafranin L, Lambert J, et al. Acute kidney injury in patients with newly diagnosed high-grade hematological malignancies: impact on remission and survival. 2013. Available at: www.plosone.org. Accessed April 13, 2013.

11. Cairo MS, Coiffier B, Reiter A, et al. Recommendations for the evaluation of risk and prophylaxis of tumor lysis syndrome (TLS) in adults and children with malignant diseases: an expert TLS panel consensus. Br J Haematol 2010;149:578–86.

12. McBride A, Westervelt P. Recognizing and managing the expanded risk of tumor lysis syndrome in hematologic and solid malignancies. J Hematol Oncol 2012;5: 75.

13. Jeha S, Kantarjan H, Irwin D, et al. Efficacy and safety of rasburicase, a recombinant urate oxidase (ElitekTM), in the management of malignancy-associated hyperuricemia in pediatric and adult patients: final results of a multicenter compassionate use trial. Leukemia 2005;19:34–8.

14. Rios A, Hagemeister FB. Chapter 41. The AIDS-related cancers. In: Kantarjian HM, Wolff RA, Koller CA, editors. The MD Anderson manual of medical oncology. 2nd edition. 2005. Available at: http://www.accessmedicine.com/content.aspx?aID=8313801. Accessed April 28, 2013.

15. McLaughlin P, Fowler N, Liu N, et al. Chapter 7. The indolent lymphomas. In: Kantarjian HM, Wolff RA, Koller CA, editors. The MD Anderson manual of medical oncology. 2nd edition. 2011. Available at: http://www.accessmedicine.com/content.aspx?aID=8301404. Accessed April 30, 2013.

16. Dunn R, Foot N, Ffolkes L, et al. Transformation form follicular lymphoma to biphasic high-grade large B-cell lymphoma with immunophenotypically and genetically distinct diffuse large B cell and Burkitt-like components. J Clin Pathol 2013;66:357–60.

17. Scholzen T, Gerdes J. The Ki-67 protein: from the known and the unknown. J Cell Physiol 2000;182(3):311–22.

18. Sehn LH, Donalsdosn J, Chhanabhai M, et al. Introduction of combined CHOP plus rituximab therapy dramatically improved outcome of diffuse large B-cell lymphoma in British Columbia. J Clin Oncol 2005;23(22):5027–33.

19. Al-Tourah AJ, Gill KK, Chhanabhai M, et al. Population-based analysis of incidence and outcome of transformed non-Hodgkin's lymphoma. J Clin Oncol 2008;26(32):5165–9.
20. Solal-Celigny P, Pascal R, Colombat P, et al. Follicular lymphoma international prognostic index. Blood 2004;104:1258–65.
21. The international non-hodgkin's lymphoma prognostic factors project. N Engl J Med 1993;329:987–94.
22. Villa D, Crump M, Panzarella T, et al. Autologous and allogeneic stem-cell transplantation for transformed follicular lymphoma: a special report of the Canadian Blood and Marrow Transplant Group. J Clin Oncol 2013;31(9):1164–71.
23. Rosen ST, Winter JN, Gordon LI, et al. Non-Hodgkin lymphoma. In: Pazdur R, Coia L, Hoskins WJ, et al, editors. Cancer Management: A Multidisciplinary Approach. 10th Edition. Lawrence, KS: CMPMedica; 2007.
24. Hehn T, Grogan TM, Miller TP. Utility of fine-needle aspiration as a diagnostic technique in lymphoma. J Clin Oncol 2004;22(15):3046–52.
25. Kinehan PE, Fletcher JW. PET/CT standardized uptake values (SUVs) in clinical practice and assessing response to therapy. Semin Ultrasound CT MR 2010; 31(6):496–505.
26. Tsuchiya KD. Fluorescence in situ hybridization. Clin Lab Med 2011;31(4): 525–42.
27. Friedberg JW. Double-hit diffuse large b-cell lymphoma. J Clin Oncol 2012; 30(28):3439–43.
28. Motillo C, Grau J, Junca J, et al. Translocation (3;8)(q27;q24) in two cases of triple hit lymphoma. Cancer Genet Cytogenet 2010;203(2):328–32.

Chronic Leukemia

Edythe M. (Lyn) Greenberg, PhD, RN, FNP-BC*,
Alexandra Probst, MS, PA-C

KEYWORDS

- Chronic myeloid leukemia • Chronic lymphocytic leukemia • Leukocytosis
- Lymphocytosis • Tyrosine kinase inhibitors • Alkylating agents
- Monoclonal antibodies • Immunomodulatory agents

KEY POINTS

- Chronic myeloid leukemia is a myeloproliferative hematopoietic stem-cell disorder of mature white blood cells of myeloid lineage.
- Chronic lymphocytic leukemia is a monoclonal B-cell disorder.
- Chronic myeloid leukemia is treated with the tyrosine kinase inhibitors.
- Front-line treatment of chronic lymphocytic leukemia includes alkylating agents, purine analogues, monoclonal antibodies, and immunomodulatory medications.

INTRODUCTION

Approximately 1 in 74 men and women will be diagnosed with leukemia during their lifetime, with chronic leukemias accounting for 45% of new leukemia cases.[1] Typically, chronic leukemias are not immediately life threatening and are classified by a clonal overproduction of mature white blood cells (WBCs). Chronic leukemias can be divided into 2 subsets: chronic myeloid leukemia (CML) and chronic lymphocytic leukemia (CLL).

CHRONIC MYELOID LEUKEMIA

CML is a clonal myeloproliferative hematopoietic stem-cell disorder accounting for approximately 15% of all adult leukemias.[2] The median age at diagnosis is 64 years of age, with a slight male predominance.[3] Unique to CML, the Philadelphia chromosome consists of a reciprocal translocation between the ABL gene found on chromosome 9 and the BCR gene from chromosome 22.[2] This fusion oncogene results in BCR-ABL tyrosine kinases and activation of downstream pathways, giving rise to clonal expansion of Philadelphia-positive cells.[2,3] BCR-ABL provides a survival

There is not direct financial interest with any company.
Department of Leukemia, MD Anderson Cancer Center, 1515 Holcombe Boulevard, Houston, TX 77030, USA
* Corresponding author.
E-mail address: emgreenb@mdanderson.org

advantage to CML cells by promoting proliferation and suppressing apoptosis.[4] Malignant cells accumulate and produce the characteristic features of CML.

Clinical Presentation and Diagnostic Workup

In many cases, CML patients are asymptomatic at the time of presentation, with abnormalities identified on routine laboratory tests. Some patients present with nonspecific symptoms including fevers, night sweats, weight loss, and bone pain. Splenomegaly can be found in 30% to 70% of CML patients at the time of diagnosis.[5] Laboratory abnormalities can include leukocytosis, basophilia, eosinophilia, and high platelet count. An elevated WBC count, usually exceeding 25×10^9/L, with left shift is the most common feature of the disease.[5]

Once a suspicion of CML is established, a bone marrow examination with cytogenetic and molecular testing is mandatory to confirm the diagnosis and identify the disease phase. The bone marrow is typically hypercellular with a predominance of myeloid precursors.[5] Up to 40% of patients can have some degree of myelofibrosis.[2] Cytogenetic analysis will identify the presence of the Philadelphia chromosome, validating the diagnosis of CML. Once CML is established, determining the disease phase is an important factor when considering prognosis and treatment options. Ninety percent of CML patients are diagnosed in chronic phase, with some patients presenting in more advanced stages to include accelerated or blast phase.[2] The University of Texas M.D. Anderson Cancer Center criteria for these phases are listed in **Table 1**. Only 1 criterion in the accelerated or blast phase has to be met to classify the disease in one of these more advanced stages.

For patients diagnosed in chronic phase, the median survival is approximately 4 to 5 years without tyrosine kinase inhibitor (TKI) therapy.[6] Accelerated phase is a transitional phase characterized by a decrease in maturation and a median survival of 1 to 2 years.[2] Blast-phase CML is the last and most aggressive stage of the disease, resembling an acute leukemia. The blasts can phenotypically be myeloid, lymphoid, or undifferentiated.[2] The median survival is 3 to 6 months, with lymphoid blast-phase CML patients having a slightly better prognosis than those in myeloid blast phase.[2] As the disease progresses, patients become more symptomatic, with increased anemia, thrombocytopenia, constitutional symptoms, and risk of infections.[2]

Table 1 CML phases						
	Blasts (%)	Blasts + Promyelocytes (%)	Basophils (%)	Platelets	Cytogenetics	Extramedullary Disease
Chronic Phase	0–14	<30	<20	>100,000	No clonal evolution	Not present
Accelerated Phase	15–29	≥30	≥20	<100,000 Unrelated to therapy	Clonal evolution	Not present
Blast Phase	≥30	—	—	—	With or without clonal evolution	Present

Data from Kantarjian HM, Wolff RA, Koller CA. MD Anderson manual of medical oncology. New York: McGraw-Hill; 2006. p. 1–74.

Treatment

While awaiting confirmation of the presence of the Philadelphia chromosome, hydroxyurea can be initiated for temporary control of elevated WBC counts. Once the diagnosis of CML is confirmed, TKI therapy is the mainstay of treatment. TKIs specifically inhibit the tyrosine kinase activity of the BCR-ABL oncogene and ABL kinase, which promotes apoptosis and cell death.[7] Imatinib (Gleevec) was the first TKI medication to be approved by the Food and Drug Administration, in May 2001. For therapy-naïve patients who were diagnosed in chronic phase and treated with imatinib, 83% achieved a complete cytogenetic remission with an overall 8-year survival rate of 85% and an 81% event-free survival.[5] Imatinib is overall a well-tolerated medication, with the most common Grade-1 to -2 adverse events including nausea, edema, muscle cramps, diarrhea, rash, weight gain, and fatigue.[8] Myelosuppression, specifically neutropenia, is the most common Grade-3 to -4 adverse event.[8] **Table 2** includes a definition of the 5 grades of adverse events.[9]

Nilotinib, dasatinib, and bosutinib are second-generation TKIs approved for the treatment of CML. Nilotinib and dasatinib are approved for front-line therapy for CML patients, while nilotinib, dasatinib, and bosutinib are approved for CML patients who have previously experienced imatinib resistance or intolerance. In newly diagnosed chronic-phase CML patients, dasatinib and nilotinib have been shown to be more potent, and with better responses and outcomes than imatinib.[10,11] The rate of complete cytogenetic remission after 36 months of therapy was 58% for imatinib, compared with 76% for nilotinib and 78% for dasatinib.[12] Each second-generation TKI is overall well tolerated, with a slightly different side-effect profile. Some of the more common adverse events noted with dasatinib include myelosuppression, pleural effusions, and headaches.[13] Nilotinib has the potential for myelosuppression along with rash, elevated liver enzymes, and hyperglycemia.[14] Bosutinib's side-effect profile includes diarrhea, nausea/vomiting, and potential elevation of liver enzymes.[15]

Ponatinib is a potent third-generation TKI currently approved for CML patients who have been resistant or intolerant to prior TKI therapy. In a recent study, in which greater than 94% of participants had been intolerant or resistant to at least 2 prior TKIs, 72% of chronic-phase CML patients had a major cytogenetic response, with 63% of chronic-phase CML patients achieving a cytogenetic remission.[16] Ponatinib

Table 2		
Grades of adverse events in CML		
Grade	Severity	Description
1	Mild	Asymptomatic or mild symptoms. Clinical or diagnostic observations only. Intervention not indicated
2	Moderate	Minimal, local, or noninvasive intervention indicated. Limiting age-appropriate instrumental activities of daily living (ADL)
3	Severe	Medically significant but not immediately life-threatening Hospitalization or prolongation of hospitalization indicated. Disabling or limiting self-care ADL
4	Life-threatening	Urgent intervention indicated, otherwise immediately life-threatening
5	Death	Death related to adverse event

Data from Kantarjian H, Shah N, Cortes J, et al. Dasatinib or imatinib in newly diagnosed chronic-phase chronic myeloid leukemia: 2-year follow-up from a randomized phase 3 trial (DASISION). Blood 2012;119:1123–9.

was also shown to be effective in CML patients who develop the T315i BCR-ABL kinase mutation, which is highly resistant to all other commercially available TKIs.[16]

Once TKI therapy has been initiated, routine laboratory tests and follow-up are necessary to monitor for response and adverse events. A repeat bone marrow examination with cytogenetic and molecular testing is typically performed every 3 to 6 months for the first 12 months or until a cytogenetic remission has been achieved.[17] Disease-response definitions and monitoring guidelines, as per the European LeukemiaNet, are given in **Table 3**.[18] A suboptimal response is defined as failing to achieve a major cytogenetic response within 6 months of therapy, or failure to achieve a cytogenetic remission within 12 months of therapy. A suboptimal response or loss of response to treatment would be an indication to consider switching to an alternative TKI.

In summary, CML is a chronic leukemia characterized by the Philadelphia chromosome, resulting in clonal myeloproliferation. Most patients are asymptomatic at the time of diagnosis, and will require a bone marrow evaluation to confirm the presence of the Philadelphia chromosome as well as to identify the disease phase. For the 90% of CML patients diagnosed in chronic phase, the standard treatment is TKI therapy. Most CML patients respond well to TKIs and go on to live full productive lives despite their diagnosis of leukemia.

CHRONIC LYMPHOCYTIC LEUKEMIA

CLL, like CML, is a disease of mature WBCs. CLL is an indolent, monoclonal disorder associated with the progressive accumulation of functionally incompetent mature B-cell lymphocytes.[19] CLL constitutes approximately 20% of all leukemias in the United States, and is the most common leukemia in Western societies.[20,21] In the United States, Asian-Pacific Islanders and Blacks have a much lower incidence of CLL than Whites.[22] CLL also has a low incidence in Asian societies, such as Japan, Korea, and China.[19] CLL increases in incidence with age, with the majority of patients being older than 50 years at the time of diagnosis.[20] Two times more males than females are diagnosed with CLL. There are no environmental factors, such as ionizing radiation or toxic chemical exposure, which predispose an individual to CLL. It is suspected that CLL can be linked to genetic factors. Approximately 20% of individuals with CLL may have a family member with CLL or another lymphoid cancer.[19,21]

Table 3
Response definitions and monitoring guidelines for CML

	Hematologic Response	Cytogenetic Response	Molecular Response
Definition	Complete: WBC <10 × 10⁹/L, platelets <450 × 10⁹/L, <5% basophils and absence of immature granulocytes, nonpalpable spleen	Complete: 0% Ph+ cells Major: 1%–35% Ph+ cells Minor: 36%–65% Ph+ cells	Major: BCR-ABL <0.1% (as per the International Scale) Complete: undetectable BCR-ABL
Monitoring	Every 2 wk until complete response achieved, then every 3 mo	Every 3–6 mo until cytogenetic remission achieved and then every 6–12 mo	Every 3 mo

Abbreviations: Ph+, Philadelphia chromosome positive; WBC, white blood cells.
Data from Baccarani M, Saglio G, Goldman J, et al. Evolving concepts in the management of chronic myeloid leukemia: recommendations from an expert panel on behalf of the European LeukemiaNet. Blood 2006;108:1809–20.

Other diseases, such as hairy cell leukemia, mantle cell lymphoma, marginal zone lymphoma, and follicular lymphoma, often can masquerade as CLL.[23] A similar monoclonal B-cell neoplasm is small lymphocytic leukemia (SLL), an indolent non-Hodgkin lymphoma. SLL involves the lymph nodes and/or spleen, but has fewer than 5000 K/µL circulating lymphocytes in the peripheral blood.[23,24] Monoclonal B-cell lymphocytosis (MBL) has an elevated clonal B-lymphocyte count in the peripheral blood, but no lymphadenopathy, organomegaly, cytopenias, or clinical symptoms.[23-25] MBL may be a precursor to CLL.[25]

Clinical Presentation and Diagnostic Workup

The diagnosis of CLL is a clinical diagnosis. Individuals with CLL can present with indolent disease or fulminant disease. Early disease may be identified when the WBC count is elevated (leukocytosis), and the absolute lymphocyte count is greater than or equal to 5,000 µL (lymphocytosis). The individual may be asymptomatic for years before a routine complete blood cell count with differential identifies the leukocytosis and lymphocytosis. In the review of systems, the individual may identify "B" symptoms, which include unintentional weight loss, fever, drenching night sweats without evidence of infection, and extreme fatigue. These individuals may have an exaggerated response to insect stings and bites. Depending on the stage of the CLL, the individual can also present with splenomegaly, hepatomegaly, skin lesions, and lymphadenopathy.[19]

A workup for CLL will include peripheral blood for a complete blood cell count and differential; a comprehensive metabolic panel; immunoglobulins; direct antiglobulin test (DAT); testing for human immunodeficiency virus, hepatitis B, and hepatitis C; and a β2-microglobulin. In addition to an elevated lymphocyte count, the lactate dehydrogenase and β2-microglobulin may be elevated. Usually all of the immunoglobulins (IgG, IgM, IgA) are low (hypogammaglobulinemia), especially in advanced disease.[19,20] A chest radiograph may be included in the workup to evaluate for lymphadenopathy and infection. The physical examination includes measurements of the superficial lymph nodes (cervical, supraclavicular, infraclavicular, axillary, and inguinal), spleen, and liver.[19] Counseling men and women on fertility options and the possible effects of treatment on their fertility is also recommended.

A bone marrow aspiration and biopsy is not necessary to make the diagnosis of CLL, but may identify factors that influence cytopenias.[20,23] It is recommended to perform a bone marrow aspiration and biopsy before initiating treatment, and to reevaluate the bone marrow if cytopenias persist after treatment.[23] The bone marrow can have 1 of 3 patterns: nodular, interstitial, or a diffuse pattern, which is seen in advanced disease. With a diffuse pattern the majority of bone marrow is replaced with hematopoietic cells and fat cells, and indicates advanced disease.[19] On the bone marrow aspiration, at least 30% of the cells should be lymphocytes to confirm the diagnosis of CLL.[23]

A CLL panel, fluorescent in situ hybridization (FISH), and conventional cytogenetics are obtained on the bone marrow or peripheral blood. In CLL, the monoclonal B cells express the CD5 cell marker commonly found on T lymphocytes.[20,23] CLL cells are also identified by B-cell surface markers including CD19, CD20, and CD23. The surface immunoglobulins, CD20 and CD79b, are expressed in lower levels than are normal B cells. Each clone of B cells expresses either κ- or λ-immunoglobulin light chains.[23]

Morphologically, the lymphocytes are small and mature with a narrow border of cytoplasm.[23] "Smudge" cells or cellular debris are identified when fragile lymphocytes are spread onto a slide.[19-21] The leukemic lymphocytes may occasionally be mixed with large, atypical lymphocytes known as prolymphocytes. More than 55% prolymphocytes in the blood confirms a diagnosis of prolymphocytic leukemia.[20,23]

Conventional cytogenetics can detect abnormalities in approximately 56% of individuals with CLL.[26] Conventional cytogenetic techniques grow CLL cells in a culture and require prompting of the cells to divide with B-cell mitogens. FISH identifies chromosomal abnormalities on dividing cells, and can identify up to 80% of molecular abnormalities.[20] The most common cytogenetic pattern with the most favorable prognosis is the deletion found on the long arm of chromosome 13. Trisomy 12 and a rare cytogenetic abnormality on the long arm of chromosome 6 have intermediate risk features.[26]

The high-risk cytogenetic abnormalities include deletions on the long arm of chromosome 11 and the short arm of chromosome 17. The tumor-suppressor protein 53 (tp53) is located on the short arm of chromosome 17. The tp53 gene is more commonly identified in individuals with progressive and refractory disease. The ataxia telangiectasia mutated (ATM) gene may be located on chromosome 11q. Deletions 17p and 11q are associated with a more aggressive disease, poor overall survival rate, and resistance to traditional chemotherapeutic treatments.[26]

CLL Staging

CLL can be staged in one of two ways, the Rai staging system and the Binet staging system. The criteria for the Rai staging system are listed in **Table 4** and those of the Binet system in **Table 5**. The two staging methods have several disadvantages. Both methods evaluate the individual only at a single point in time, do not predict who will have disease progression, and do not determine which individuals will respond to treatment.[21,23,26]

Other Prognostic Indicators

Other clinical prognostic indicators are available to determine individuals at high risk for disease progression, a shorter time to treatment, and poorer prognosis. These indicators include a short lymphocyte doubling time, a positive Zeta alpha protein (ZAP-70), positive CD38, somatic mutation in the immunoglobulin heavy-chain variable region genes (IgVH), an increased β2-microglobulin level, diffuse pattern of bone marrow infiltration, advanced age, and an increased number of prolymphocytes. A short lymphocyte doubling time is defined as the amount of time it takes for the lymphocyte count to double. A rapid doubling time within 12 months is associated

Table 4 Rai staging of CLL		
Rai Stage	**Modified Rai Staging**	**Criteria**
0	Low risk	Elevated lymphocyte count $\geq 5 \times 10^9$
1	Intermediate risk	Elevated lymphocyte count $\geq 5 \times 10^9$ Enlarged lymph nodes
2	Intermediate risk	Elevated lymphocyte count $\geq 5 \times 10^9$ Enlarged spleen or liver with or without enlarged lymph nodes
3	High risk	Elevated lymphocyte count $\geq 5 \times 10^9$ and hemoglobin <11 g/dL
4	High risk	Elevated lymphocyte count $\geq 5 \times 10^9$ and platelet count <100 × 10^9/L

Data from Refs.[21,24,25]

Table 5 Binet staging of CLL		
Binet Staging	**Risk**	**Criteria**
A	Low	Up to 2 areas of enlarged lymph nodes >1 cm in diameter Platelets >100 × 10^9/L Hemoglobin ≥10 g/dL
B	Intermediate	≥3 areas of enlarged lymph nodes >1 cm in diameter Platelets >100 × 10^9/L Hemoglobin ≥10 g/dL
C	High	Any number of enlarged lymph nodes >1 cm in diameter Platelets <100 × 10^9/L Hemoglobin <10 g/dL

Areas of lymph node involvement:
1. Head and neck, including Waldeyer ring
2. Axillae
3. Groin
4. Palpable spleen
5. Palpable liver

Data from Desai S, Pinilla-Ibarz J. Front-line therapy for chronic lymphocytic leukemia. Cancer Control 2012;19:26–36; and Sagatys EM, Zhang L. Clinical and laboratory prognostic indicators in chronic lymphocytic leukemia. Cancer Control 2012;19:18–25.

with a shorter mean survival time.[23,26] These clinical prognostic indicators can help identify a CLL patient who is at high risk for disease progression and who may need early treatment.

Flow cytometry calculates ZAP-70 and the cell surface glycoprotein, CD38. ZAP70 signals T cells, but is abnormally expressed on malignant B cells. ZAP-70 is considered positive when more than 20% of the B cells express ZAP-70 in their cytoplasm. CD38 is considered positive when more than 30% of the B cells demonstrate CD38 in their cytoplasm. Individuals with a positive ZAP-70 and CD38 have a poorer overall survival rate.[23,26]

Leukemic cells express immunoglobulin, which may have a somatic mutation in the IgVH. The IgVH is defined as greater than a 2% deviation from the germline nucleotide sequence. An IgVH value greater than or equal to 2% deviation from the germline sequence indicates mutation. Individuals with a mutated IgVH have a better survival rate.[26]

β2-Microglobulin is a component of the human leukocyte antigen (HLA) class 1 molecules, which are located on all nucleated cells with the exception of red blood cells. A β2-microglobulin level of less than 3.5 mg/L typically indicates a greater length of time to progression of CLL. A higher β2-microglobulin level is associated with lower rates of complete remission and a shorter overall survival rate. Because β2-microglobulin can also increase with renal disease, an adjustment in the β2-microglobulin level should be made based on the glomerular filtration rate.[26]

Thymidine kinase (TK) is a protein involved in DNA synthesis. An increase in TK of greater than 7.0 U/L in an individual with early CLL can indicate a potential for more aggressive disease.[26]

Complications of CLL

Individuals with CLL have a defect in their immune systems that can result in an increased incidence of autoimmune hemolytic anemia, autoimmune thrombocytopenia, and infections. Autoimmune hemolytic anemia in CLL may present with a positive direct antiglobulin (Coombs) test (DAT), a decrease in hemoglobin, an increased reticulocyte count, elevated indirect bilirubin, or elevated lactate dehydrogenase (LDH).[27,28] When the bone marrow is heavily infiltrated with CLL, the DAT can be negative despite hemolysis, and there may not be an increase in the reticulocyte count. The LDH may also be elevated from disease progression, changes in the CLL, and liver dysfunction.[27] The serum bilirubin may not increase if the liver is able to metabolize the bilirubin.[27] Moreover, the haptoglobulin level will be low.[27,28]

In autoimmune thrombocytopenia associated with CLL, there is a rapid decrease in the platelet count. The bone marrow produces an adequate amount of megakaryocytes, but the peripheral blood platelet count remains low. The platelet count is usually less than or equal to 50,000/μL.[28] Front-line treatment includes steroids or intravenous immunoglobulin (IVIG), followed by rituximab in refractory disease.[28]

Patients with CLL are immunosuppressed, and therefore should be monitored for opportunistic infections such as fungal infections (ie, *Pneumocystis carinii* pneumonia and *Aspergillus* pneumonia); bacterial infections (ie, *Haemophilus influenzae*, *Staphylococcus aureus*, and *Streptococcus pneumoniae*); and viral infections (ie, herpes zoster). CLL patients respond well to antibiotics.[19,28] Many CLL patients will develop a hypogammaglobulinemia during their illness. Low levels of immunoglobulin G are associated with an increased incidence of bacterial infections such as *Streptococcus pneumoniae* and *Haemophilus influenzae*. Prophylactic IVIG may be beneficial when levels of immunoglobulin G are low.[19,28]

Patients with CLL may also develop secondary malignancies such as squamous cell carcinoma, melanomas, colon cancer, lung cancer, and therapy-related acute myeloid leukemia/myelodysplastic syndrome.[19] CLL can also transform into an aggressive large B-cell lymphoma known as Richter transformation.[19]

Front-Line Treatment of CLL

The decision to initiate treatment is determined by the clinical presentation of the individual. Early stage disease (Rai stage 0–1 or Binet A) in asymptomatic individuals can be managed with observation and monitoring blood counts until the disease progresses.[21] Individuals with intermediate-risk or high-risk disease (Rai stage 2–4 or Binet B and C) may benefit from treatment. Active disease should be documented before initiating treatment. Active disease includes evidence of bone marrow progression; symptomatic splenomegaly or a spleen measuring at least 6 cm below the costal margin; large lymph nodes; a short lymphocyte doubling time; autoimmune hemolytic anemia or thrombocytopenia; symptomatic anemia and/or thrombocytopenia; and "B" symptoms, including significant fatigue, fevers for 2 or more weeks without any evidence of infection, or drenching night sweats for at least 1 month or recurrent infections.[20,21,23]

If treatment is indicated, chemotherapy options include purine analogues (fludarabine, pentostatin, cladribine), alkylating agents (chlorambucil, bendamustine, cyclophosphamide), monoclonal antibodies (rituximab, ofatumumab, alemtuzumab), or a combination of these agents.[20] Alkylator-based therapy, chlorambucil, was the first medication used in the treatment of CLL.[20,21] Single-agent chlorambucil or when used in combination with corticosteroids was not proved to increase survival rate.[20] With the introduction of newer therapies, chlorambucil has limited uses but may be effective in the older adult with a poor performance status, because it has fewer adverse side effects, is rapidly absorbed from the gastrointestinal tract, and is inexpensive.[21]

In the 1990s, fludarabine was proved to improve the overall survival of CLL patients in comparison with chlorambucil. Fludarabine combined with cyclophosphamide has demonstrated better complete response rates and a longer duration of remission.[20,28] Individuals who were not refractory to fludarabine had a better overall response rate (80%) when compared with individuals who were refractory to fludarabine (38%).[29]

With the discovery of monoclonal antibodies, the combination of fludarabine, cyclophosphamide, and rituximab (FCR) became front-line treatment for CLL. Rituximab, a monoclonal antibody, affects CD20, which can be identified in mature B-cell malignancies, and improves response rates in CLL when given in high doses, frequently, or administered early in the disease.[21,30] Rituximab may sensitize CLL cells to fludarabine. In 1999, investigators from M.D. Anderson Cancer Center treated 300 individuals with FCR.[30] At 6 years, the overall survival rate was 77%.[31] However, in older adults (≥65 years), the FCR regimen may be too toxic because of myelosuppression and infection. Tolerance to FCR may be dependent on physiologic fitness rather than chronologic age. In older adults, FCR may be administered with a reduced dosage or a fewer number of cycles.[30]

Pentostatin may be substituted for fludarabine, and when administered with cyclophosphamide and rituximab (PCR) may have a lower toxicity in individuals intolerant to the FCR regimen. However, PCR's overall response rate is lower than that of FCR.[30] Bendamustine combined with rituximab is also a less toxic alternative to fludarabine, but has a complete remission rate lower than that of FCR.[30] Bendamustine has also shown efficacy in refractory or relapsed CLL patients.[20,30]

Alemtuzumab is a humanized monoclonal antibody that affects CD52, which is a cell marker expressed on both B-cell and T-cell lymphocytes. Alemtuzumab is effective in fludarabine-resistant disease or high-risk disease such as deletion 17p/tp53, and has been combined with FCR (CFAR) in both front-line treatment and relapsed/refractory disease.[30] Alemtuzumab is myelosuppressive, which can result in opportunistic infections such as reactivation of the cytomegalovirus (CMV), *Pneumocystis jiroveci* pneumonia, herpes simplex virus, *Listeria monocytogenes*, and *Aspergillus* pneumonia.[30] Any individual treated with alemtuzumab should receive prophylaxis antibiotics for CMV and pneumocytic pneumonia.

Ofatumumab, a humanized monoclonal antibody, is currently being investigated as both front-line therapy and in relapsed/refractory disease. Single-agent rituximab and ofatumumab are less myelosuppressive.[30] Most commonly the monoclonal antibodies are associated with transfusion reactions such as hypotension and chills.

Immunomodulatory medications such as lenalidomide have been used both as single agents and in combination with monoclonal antibodies to treat CLL. In a 2011 study, participants who included adults 65 years and older received lenalidomide 5 mg, which was titrated up to 25 mg as tolerated.[32] Treatment was continued until the CLL progressed. More than 65% of the participants achieved a response, including a 10% complete response rate, 5% complete response with residual cytopenias, 7% nodular response, and 43% partial response. The most common adverse event was neutropenia.[32]

Lenalidomide has been associated with tumor flare syndrome, rashes, fatigue, myelosuppression, and embolic phenomenon. Tumor flare syndrome is most commonly seen in patients with large lymph nodes, and occurs when the lymph nodes become larger before shrinking in size. Individuals treated with lenalidomide are at risk for embolic phenomenon such as deep vein thrombosis and pulmonary emboli. If myelosuppression occurs, the dosage of the lenalidomide may be reduced.[33]

At present, allogeneic hematopoietic stem-cell transplantation (SCT) is the only option for a potential cure for chronic lymphocytic leukemia.[34] Hematopoietic SCT evaluation is recommended for younger individuals with CLL and high-risk features such as deletion 17p/tp53 and deletion 11q/ATM.[20] Autologous SCT may lead to a good response rate, but has a high association with relapse. Allogeneic SCT may produce a durable remission but is associated with higher toxicities.[20] New treatments are being investigated, including the Bruton tyrosine kinase (BTK) inhibitors, BH-3 mimetics, Syk inhibitors, inhibitors of phosphatidylinositol-3-kinase, and CD37.[20]

Response to Treatment

Individuals are considered to be in complete remission when they have an absolute lymphocyte count of less than 5000; lymph nodes measuring less than 1.5 cm; no splenomegaly or hepatomegaly; no "B" symptoms; and no cytopenias as evidenced by an absolute neutrophil count greater than 1500/μL; platelet count greater than 100,000/μL; and hemoglobin greater than 11.0 g. No minimal residual disease should be present on flow cytometry. Partial remission is defined by a 50% decrease in the absolute lymphocyte count; a reduction in lymphadenopathy; a reduction by 50% of pretreatment liver or spleen size by palpation or computed tomography scan; and at least 1 of the following: blood counts including an absolute neutrophil count greater than 1500/μL, platelet count greater than 100,000/μL or a 50% improvement of baseline, or hemoglobin greater than 11.0 g or a 50% improvement over baseline. CLL is considered to have progressed when there is enlargement of lymph nodes; new organomegaly or an increase in the size of the liver or spleen by 50%; a 50% increase in the absolute lymphocyte count; and cytopenias. In a patient who has obtained a complete or partial remission, relapsed disease is present if the symptoms of disease reappear 6 or more months after treatment. Refractory disease is defined as disease progression or treatment failure within 6 months of the chemoimmunotherapy.[23]

SUMMARY

The chronic leukemias are diseases of mature WBCs. CML is a myeloproliferative hematopoietic stem-cell disorder of mature WBCs of myeloid lineage, and CLL is a monoclonal B-cell disorder. Over the last decade, new therapies have been developed for the treatment of these disorders. With the advent of new therapies, individuals with chronic leukemia are living much longer and are leading fulfilling lives.

REFERENCES

1. National Cancer Institute. SEER stat facts: leukemia. 2009. Available at: http://seer.cancer.gov/statfacts/html/leuks.html. Accessed March 21, 2013.
2. Kantarjian HM, Wolff RA, Koller CA. MD Anderson manual of medical oncology. New York: McGraw-Hill; 2006. p. 1–74.
3. National Cancer Institute. SEER stat facts: chronic myeloid leukemia. 2009. Available at: http://seer.cancer.gov/statfacts/html/cmyl.html. Accessed January 31, 2013.
4. Kantarjian H, Giles F, Quintas-Cardama A, et al. Important therapeutic targets in chronic myelogenous leukemia. Clin Cancer Res 2007;13:1089.
5. Cortes J, Silver R, Kantarjian H. Chronic myeloid leukemia. Cancer Network; 2011. Available at: http://www.cancernetwork.com/cancer-management/chronic-myeloid-leukemia/article/10165/1802798. Accessed February 7, 2013.
6. Cortes J, Kantarjian H. How I treat newly diagnosed chronic phase CML. Blood 2012;120:1390–7.
7. Woessner D, Lim C. Disrupting BCR-ABL in combination with secondary leukemia-specific pathways in CML cells leads to enhanced apoptosis and decreased proliferation. Mol Pharm 2013;10:270–7.

8. Baccarani M, Druker B, Cortes-Franco J, et al. 24 Months update of the TOPS study. Blood (ASH Annual Meeting Abstracts) 2009;114 [abstract 337].
9. National Cancer Institute. NCI guidelines for investigators: adverse event reporting requirements. Available at: http://ctep.cancer.gov/protocolDevelopment/electronic_applications/docs/aeguidelines.pdf. Accessed February 29, 2013.
10. Kantarjian H, Shah N, Cortes J, et al. Dasatinib or imatinib in newly diagnosed chronic-phase chronic myeloid leukemia: 2-year follow-up from a randomized phase 3 trial (DASISION). Blood 2012;119:1123–9.
11. Kantarjian H, Hochhaus A, Saglio G, et al. Nilotinib versus imatinib for the treatment of patients with newly diagnosed chronic phase, Philadelphia chromosome-positive, chronic myeloid leukaemia: 24-month minimum follow-up of the phase 3 randomised ENESTnd trial. Lancet Oncol 2011;12:841–51.
12. Alattar M, Kantarjian H, Jabbour E, et al. Clinical significance of complete cytogenetic response (CCyR) and major molecular response (MMR) achieved with different treatment modalities used as frontline therapy in chronic myeloid leukemia (CML) chronic phase. Blood (ASH Annual Meeting Abstracts) 2011;118 [abstract 745].
13. Kantarjian H, Shah N, Hochhaus A, et al. Dasatinib versus imatinib in newly diagnosed chronic-phase chronic myeloid leukemia. N Engl J Med 2010;362: 2260–70.
14. Saglio G, Kim D, Issaragrisil S, et al. Nilotinib versus imatinib in newly diagnosed chronic-phase chronic myeloid leukemia. N Engl J Med 2010;362: 2251–9.
15. Cortes J, Kim D, Kantarjian H, et al. Bosutinib versus imatinib in newly diagnosed chronic-phase chronic myeloid leukemia: results from the BELA Trial. J Clin Oncol 2012;30:3486–92.
16. Cortes J, Kantarjian H, Shah N, et al. Ponatinib in refractory Philadelphia chromosome-positive leukemias. N Engl J Med 2012;367:2075–88.
17. Jabbour E, Cortes J, Kantarjian H. Molecular monitoring in chronic myeloid leukemia. Cancer 2012;112:2112–8.
18. Baccarani M, Saglio G, Goldman J, et al. Evolving concepts in the management of chronic myeloid leukemia: recommendations from an expert panel on behalf of the European LeukemiaNet. Blood 2006;108:1809–20.
19. Kipps K. Chronic lymphocytic leukemia and related diseases. In: Kaushansky K, Lichtman MA, Beutler E, et al, editors. Williams hematology. 8th edition. New York: McGraw Hill Medical; 2010. p. 1431–81.
20. Garg RJ, Bueso-Ramos CE, O'Brien S. Chronic lymphocytic leukemia and associated disorders. In: Kantarjian HM, Wolff RA, Koller CA, editors. MD Anderson manual of medical oncology. New York: The McGraw-Hill Medical Publishing Division; 2011. p. 33–52.
21. Desai S, Pinilla-Ibarz J. Front-line therapy for chronic lymphocytic leukemia. Cancer Control 2012;19:26–36.
22. Yamamoto JF, Goodman MT. Patterns of leukemia incidence in the United States by subtype and demographic characteristics, 1997-2001. Cancer Causes Control 2008;19:379–90.
23. Halleck M, Cheson BD, Catovsky D, et al. Guidelines for the diagnosis and treatment of chronic lymphocytic leukemia: a report from the International Workshop on Chronic Lymphocytic Leukemia updating the National Cancer Institute-Working Group 1996 guidelines. Blood 2008;111:5446–54.
24. Sagatys EM, Zhang L. Clinical and laboratory prognostic indicators in chronic lymphocytic leukemia. Cancer Control 2012;19:18–25.

25. Mowery YM, Lanasa MC. Clinical aspects of monoclonal B-cell lymphocytosis. Cancer Control 2012;19:8.
26. Mougalian SS, O'Brien S. Adverse prognostic features in chronic lymphocytic leukemia. Oncology 2011;258:692–702.
27. Packman CH. Hemolytic anemia resulting from immune injury. In: Kaushansky K, Lichtman MA, Beutler E, et al, editors. Williams hematology. 8th edition. New York: McGraw Hill Medical; 2010. p. 777–98.
28. Dearden C. Disease-specific complications of chronic lymphocytic leukemia. Hematology Am Soc Hematol Educ Program 2008;2008:450–6.
29. O'Brien SM, Kantarjian HM, Cortes J, et al. Results of the fludarabine and cyclophosphamide combination regimen in chronic lymphocytic leukemia. J Clin Oncol 2001;19:1414–20.
30. Tam CS, Keating MJ. Chemoimmunotherapy of chronic lymphocytic leukemia. Nat Rev Clin Oncol 2010;7:521–32.
31. Tam CS, O'Brien S, Wierfa W, et al. Long-term results of the fludarabine cyclophosphamide, and rituximab regimen as initial therapy of chronic leukemia. Blood 2008;9:975–80.
32. Badoux XC, Keating MJ, Wen S, et al. Lenalidomide as initial therapy of elderly patients with chronic lymphocytic leukemia. Blood 2011;118:3489–98.
33. Carballido E, Veliz M, Komrokji R, et al. Immunomodulatory drugs and active immunotherapy for chronic lymphocytic leukemia. Cancer Control 2012;19:54–67.
34. Karfan-Dabaja MA, Bazarbachi A. Hematopoietic stem cell allografting for chronic lymphocytic leukemia: a focus on reduced-intensity conditioning regimens. Cancer Control 2012;19:68–75.

Management of Anticoagulation in the Critically Ill Patient

Katy M. Toale, PharmD, BCPS

KEYWORDS

- Anticoagulation • Anticoagulant protocols • Heparin
- Low-molecular-weight heparin • Direct thrombin inhibitors • Bleeding

KEY POINTS

- Anticoagulation is often used in the intensive care unit for indications such as venous thromboembolism treatment and prophylaxis, acute coronary syndrome, atrial fibrillation, and heparin-induced thrombocytopenia.
- The most commonly used anticoagulation agents are heparin and low-molecular-weight heparins.
- Low-molecular-weight heparins have a favorable pharmacokinetic and adverse effect profile and the anticoagulation effect is more predictable; however, heparin is often preferred because of its shorter half-life and ability to be completely reversed in the setting of bleeding or the need for an urgent procedure.
- Direct thrombin inhibitors can be used for patients with heparin-induced thrombocytopenia or potentially as an alternative to traditional therapies in percutaneous coronary interventions.

INTRODUCTION

Anticoagulation is often needed in the critically ill patient for many reasons including prevention and treatment of venous thromboembolism (VTE), acute coronary syndrome (ACS), atrial fibrillation, and heparin-induced thrombocytopenia (HIT). The agent most often used is heparin because of its short half-life and the availability of a reversal agent. Protocols are needed because of the difficulty in dosing and monitoring of these agents, and nurse-driven protocols play an essential role in management.

HEPARIN

For many decades, heparin has been available as an anticoagulant for use in the intensive care unit (ICU). Heparin works by binding to antithrombin, which then inactivates

Disclosures: None.
Department of Pharmacy, MD Anderson Cancer Center, 1515 Holcombe Boulevard, Unit 377, Houston, TX 77030, USA
E-mail address: khanzelka@mdanderson.org

Crit Care Nurs Clin N Am 25 (2013) 471–480
http://dx.doi.org/10.1016/j.ccell.2013.08.002
0899-5885/13/$ – see front matter
© 2013 Elsevier Inc. All rights reserved.

primarily thrombin (factor IIa) and factor Xa (**Fig. 1**). As a result, heparin prevents fibrin formation and inhibits activation of platelets.[1]

Because heparin is a mixture of molecules that vary in length, the anticoagulant effect can vary from patient to patient. Another disadvantage of heparin is that it is highly protein bound, which can make the anticoagulation effects unpredictable. Heparin is a large molecule; therefore, it is unable to bind to clot-bound thrombin (**Fig. 2**). Clot-bound thrombin maintains the ability to activate the coagulation cascade, which could be detrimental to the patient. Heparin can only inactivate the clotting process; it does not lyse blood clots.[2]

Dosing

Heparin infusions are dosed based on the indication for treatment of VTE, ACS, or VTE prophylaxis, and the recommended dosages are presented in **Box 1**. Controversies exist on whether heparin should be used in the acute management of ischemic stroke. With the current evidence available, urgent anticoagulation is not recommended for management of acute ischemic stroke.[3] Originally, heparin infusions used standard dosing scales; however, research has shown that weight-based dosing is superior in achieving therapeutic anticoagulation.[4,5] Nurse-driven protocols allow safe and effective titration of heparin to achieve therapeutic anticoagulation in a timelier manner. Examples of dosing protocols used at our institution are presented in **Figs. 3** and **4**. The half-life of heparin can vary based on the dosage administered. Half-life variability occurs because initial doses of heparin are rapidly cleared through a saturable process. Once these mechanisms are saturated, the elimination of heparin is much slower. As a result, larger bolus doses result in a longer half-life of the medication and could potentially result in supratherapeutic anticoagulation.[2]

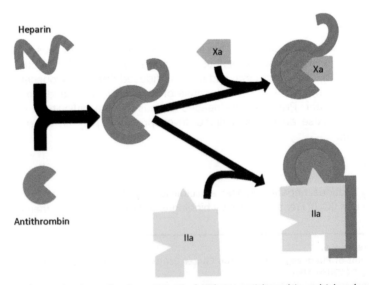

Fig. 1. Heparin mechanism of action. Heparin binds to antithrombin, which subsequently binds to and inactivates thrombin (factor IIa) and Xa. Inhibition of thrombin requires heparin chain lengths of at least 18 saccharide units. LMWHs are generally not large enough to bind thrombin; therefore they have greater activity against factor Xa.

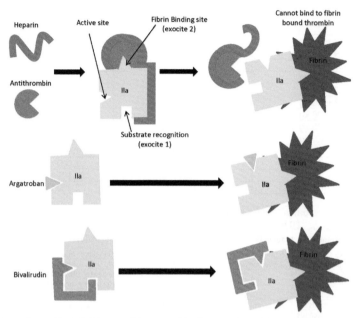

Fig. 2. Direct thrombin inhibitor and heparin binding to thrombin and fibrin. Heparin binds to antithrombin, which subsequently binds to and inactivates thrombin (factor IIa). The heparin/antithrombin complex is unable to bind to clot-bound thrombin. Argatroban binds to the active site and bivalirudin binds to the active site and exosite 1, which allow them to inhibit free-floating thrombin as well as fibrin-bound thrombin.

Monitoring

Because of the pharmacokinetic disadvantages discussed earlier, which result in unpredictable responses in patients, heparin infusions must be monitored to ensure an adequate anticoagulation effect. The 2 most common laboratory tests used to monitor heparin are the activated partial thromboplastin time (aPTT) and antifactor

---

Box 1
Dosing of heparin

Venous thromboembolism treatment

1. Initial 80 units/kg IV bolus followed by 18 units/kg/h IV continuous infusion

2. Initial 333 units/kg SC followed by 250 units/kg SC twice daily

ACS/unstable angina/atrial fibrillation

1. 60–70 units/kg (max 5000 units) IV bolus followed by 12 to 15 units/kg/h (max 1000 units/h) IV continuous infusion

2. If given in conjunction with a fibrinolytic agent: 60 units/kg (max 4500 units) IV bolus followed by 12 units/kg/h (max 1000 units/h) IV continuous infusion

Venous thromboembolism prophylaxis

1. 5000 units SC every 8 hours

Abbreviations: IV, intravenous; SC, subcutaneous.

Weight	Heparin Bolus (80 units / kg)	Initial Infusion rate (18 units / kg / hour)
47 – 53 kg	4,000 units	900 units / hour
54 – 59 kg	4,500 units	1,000 units / hour
60 – 65 kg	5,000 units	1,100 units / hour
66 – 71 kg	5,500 units	1,200 units / hour
72 – 78 kg	6,000 units	1,300 units / hour
79 – 78 kg	6,500 units	1,500 units / hour
85 – 90 kg	7,000 units	1,600 units / hour
91 – 96 kg	7,500 units	1,700 units / hour
97 – 103 kg	8,000 units	1,800 units / hour
104 – 109 kg	8,500 units	1,900 units / hour
110 – 115 kg	9,000 units	2,000 units / hour
116 – 121 kg	9,500 units	2,100 units / hour
Greater than 121 kg	10,000 units	2,200 units / hour

Heparin Dosing Scale for VTE and other High-Risk Patients (Target aPTT = heparin anti-Xa activity of 0.3 – 0.7 units/mL)			
aPTT Obtained	Bolus Dose	Infusion Hold Time	Infusion rate Change
Less than 45 seconds	5,000 units	----	Increase rate by 200 units / hour, obtain aPTT n 6 hours
45 – 59 seconds	2,500 units	----	Increase rate by 100 units / hour, obtain aPTT n 6 hours
60 – 100 seconds	----	----	Continue same rate, obtain aPTT in 6 hours
101 – 120 seconds	----	----	Decrease rate by 100 units / hour, obtain aPTT n 6 hours
121 – 140 seconds	----	30 minutes	Decrease rate by 200 units / hour, obtain aPTT n 6 hours
141 – 160 seconds	----	60 minutes	Decrease rate by 300 units / hour, obtain aPTT n 6 hours
Greater than 160 seconds	----	120 minutes	Decrease rate by 400 units / hour, obtain aPTT n 6 hours

Fig. 3. Heparin weight-based dosing for venous thromboembolism. (*Courtesy of* The University of Texas MD Anderson Cancer Center, Houston, TX. © 2010; with permission.)

Xa (anti-Xa) levels. The therapeutic interval for aPTT varies from institution to institution because the measured response to the aPTT is not standard and depends on which reagent and instrumentation is used.[1] The aPTT should be repeated every 6 hours after initiation of the heparin infusion and/or dose change. For patients undergoing percutaneous coronary intervention (PCI) or cardiopulmonary bypass surgery, which require higher doses of heparin, the activated clotting time (ACT) is used to monitor

Weight	Heparin Bolus (60 units / kg)	Initial Infusion rate (12 units / kg / hour)
47 – 53 kg	3,000 units	600 units / hour
55 – 62 kg	3,500 units	700 units / hour
63 – 70 kg	4,000 units	800 units / hour
71 – 79 kg	4,500 units	900 units / hour
Greater than 79 kg	5,000 units	1,000 units / hour

Heparin Dosing Scale for Acute Coronary Syndrome and Atrial Fibrillation (Target aPTT = 1.5 to 2.5 x control)			
aPTT Obtained	Bolus Dose	Infusion Hold Time	Infusion rate Change
Less than 30 seconds	5,000 units	----	Increase rate by 200 units / hour, obtain aPTT n 6 hours
30 – 44 seconds	2,500 units	----	Increase rate by 100 units / hour, obtain aPTT n 6 hours
45 – 75 seconds	----	----	Continue same rate, obtain aPTT in 6 hours
76 – 90 seconds	----	----	Decrease rate by 100 units / hour, obtain aPTT n 6 hours
91 – 120 seconds	----	30 minutes	Decrease rate by 200 units / hour, obtain aPTT n 6 hours
121 – 150 seconds	----	60 minutes	Decrease rate by 300 units / hour, obtain aPTT n 6 hours
Greater than 150 seconds	----	120 minutes	Decrease rate by 400 units / hour, obtain aPTT n 6 hours

Fig. 4. Heparin weight-based dosing for ACS/atrial fibrillation. (*Courtesy of* The University of Texas MD Anderson Cancer Center, Houston, TX. © 2010; with permission.)

the heparin dose.[1] Certain patients may experience heparin resistance and require unusually large doses of heparin (>35,000 units/d) to maintain a therapeutic aPTT. In these cases, anti-Xa levels should be used to guide heparin dosage adjustments, rather than aPTT levels.[1]

Adverse Effects

Heparin has the potential to interact with platelet factor 4, which can induce HIT. Although the name HIT implies a state where the patient is at risk for bleeding because of a low platelet count, the opposite is true. HIT is a prothrombotic state that can result in life-threatening thrombotic events if not treated immediately. The treatment of choice is nonheparin anticoagulants such as argatroban or bivalirudin.[6] Heparin can also result in bleeding complications, and long-term use has been associated with osteoporosis. Other rare adverse events include skin necrosis, local urticaria, and inhibition of aldosterone synthesis, which can result in hyperkalemia.[7]

Reversal

A common reason for the frequent use of heparin in the ICU setting is the availability of intravenous (IV) protamine, which can fully reverse the anticoagulant effect in patients experiencing a bleeding complication or needing an emergent procedure. The dosing of protamine depends on the dose of heparin given.[8,9] Dosing of protamine can be based on the following guidelines:

- Determine the units of heparin the patient has received in the previous 2 hours
- Divide this number by 100
  - One milligram of protamine neutralizes about 100 units of heparin
- Single doses of protamine should not exceed 50 mg and slow administration (≤5 mg/min) is recommended. Repeat doses can be administered after 10 to 15 minutes if needed
- Example: A patient is receiving 1250 units per hour of heparin. The dose of protamine should be 25 mg

Adverse reactions of protamine include hypotension, flushing, and bradycardia; however, these can be avoided by infusing protamine slowly.[1]

LOW-MOLECULAR-WEIGHT HEPARINS

Low-molecular-weight heparins (LMWHs) are smaller fragments of heparin produced from a controlled enzymatic or chemical depolymerization process. The smaller size allows for greater activity against factor Xa compared with heparin.[10] A comparison of heparin and LMWHs is presented in **Table 1**. LMWHs have less protein-binding properties and a longer half-life, therefore they have the advantage of producing a more predictable anticoagulation response compared with heparin. The use of LMWHs in an ICU setting is limited because they are predominately eliminated by the kidneys and there is no agent that can completely reverse the anticoagulant effect. Because of the high incidence of acute kidney injury in the ICU and the potential delay in increase in serum creatinine levels, LMWHs are often not the treatment of choice.

Dosing

Dosing of LMWHs for different indications can be seen in **Box 2**. Dosages of enoxaparin should be reduced for patients with a creatinine clearance (CrCl) of less than 30 mL/min and all LMWHs should be avoided if CrCl is less than 20 mL/min.

Table 1
Comparison of heparin and LMWHs

	Advantages	Disadvantages
Heparin	Short half-life: 0.5 h Completely reversed by protamine Can be used in renal insufficiency	Variability in anticoagulation effect Unable to bind and inactivate clot-bound thrombin Risk of HIT Risk of osteoporosis Coagulation monitoring necessary
LMWHs	Long half-life 3–6 h allows for easier dosing Predictable dose response Lower incidence of HIT Lower risk of osteoporosis No need for routine monitoring	Long half-life 3–6 h could be detrimental for a patient with a bleeding complication Unable to bind and inactivate clot-bound thrombin Only partially reversed by protamine Cleared primarily by the kidney and cannot be used in renal failure

Abbreviation: HIT, heparin-induced thrombocytopenia.

Monitoring

Monitoring the anticoagulation response is not routinely recommended. Clinicians may consider monitoring of anti-Xa levels for obese patients, patients with renal insufficiency, or during pregnancy. The recommended peak anti-Xa level for treatment of

Box 2
Dosing of LMWHs

Enoxaparin

1. VTE prophylaxis with hip or knee surgery: 30 mg SC every 12 hours
2. VTE prophylaxis with abdominal or colorectal surgery: 40 mg SC every 24 hours
3. VTE prophylaxis in medical patients: 40 mg SC every 24 hours
4. VTE treatment: 1 mg/kg SC twice daily or 1.5 mg/kg SC once daily
5. Unstable angina/non–Q-wave myocardial infarction: 1 mg/kg SC twice daily
6. ST-elevation myocardial infarction: initial IV bolus 30 mg then 1 mg/kg SC twice daily

Dalteparin

1. VTE prophylaxis with hip surgery: 5000 units SC daily
2. VTE prophylaxis with abdominal surgery: 5000 units SC daily
3. Unstable angina/non–Q-wave myocardial infarction: 120 units/kg SC every 12 hours
4. VTE treatment in patients who have cancer: 200 units/kg SC once daily for 30 days, then 150 units/kg SC daily

Tinzaparin

1. VTE prophylaxis with hip or knee surgery: 75 units SC daily
2. VTE prophylaxis with general surgery: 3500 units SC daily
3. VTE treatment: 175 units/kg SC daily

Abbreviations: SC, subcutaneous; VTE, venous thromboembolism.

VTE with twice daily dosing is 0.5 to 1.0 unit/mL and, for once daily dosing, is 1.0 to 2.0 units/mL. The recommended range for ACS is 0.5 to 1.5 units/mL.[11]

Adverse Effects

The adverse effects of LMWHs are similar to heparin with bleeding complications being the most common. LMWHs also have the ability to cause HIT and osteoporosis; however, the risk is much lower than with heparin.[1]

Reversal

No agent is currently available to fully reverse the anticoagulant effects of LMWHs. Protamine only partially reverses the effect because it only neutralizes factor IIa and has a partial effect on factor Xa.[9] If indicated, protamine should be prescribed as follows:

- If LMWH has been given in the previous 8 hours
  - 1 mg of protamine per 1 mg of enoxaparin or
  - 1 mg of protamine per 100 units of dalteparin/tinzaparin
- If LMWH was given greater than 8 hours ago
  - 0.5 mg of protamine per 1 mg of enoxaparin or
  - 0.5 mg of protamine per 100 units of dalteparin/tinzaparin
- Single doses of protamine should not exceed 50 mg and slow administration (≤5 mg/min) is recommended. Repeat doses can be administered after 10 to 15 minutes if needed because of the short half-life of protamine.[1]

DIRECT THROMBIN INHIBITORS

Thrombin is the central factor responsible for the final step of thrombus creation. Developing therapies to target thrombin has provided additional treatment options for anticoagulation. Because thrombin can amplify its own production and continue to activate the coagulation cascade, inhibition is crucial to the management of thromboembolic diseases.[12] Three direct thrombin inhibitors (DTIs) are currently available on the market: argatroban, bivalirudin, and dabigatran. Dabigatran has limited use in the ICU because it is an oral anticoagulant with a longer duration of action and no known reversal agent. The main indication for DTI use in the ICU is HIT; however, bivalirudin can also be used for patients with ACS undergoing PCI. DTIs do not bind to antithrombin to inactivate thrombin; they block either the active site alone or both the active site and exosite 1 to inhibit thrombin activity. The action of DTIs provides the advantage of being able to bind and inactivate clot-bound thrombin, which cannot be accomplished by heparin (see **Fig. 2**).

Dosing

Dosing for the DTIs can be seen in **Box 3**.[6] Argatroban clearance is largely affected by hepatic function. For patients in the ICU with impaired hepatic function, bivalirudin may be a better option. Bivalirudin elimination is mainly bienzymatic with a small amount cleared renally. Therefore, in severe renal dysfunction, dosing of bivalirudin should be adjusted.[13]

Monitoring

The half-life of the DTIs is short (argatroban, 40–50 minutes; bivalirudin, 25 minutes) therefore an aPTT should be obtained every 2 hours after initiation and after any dose change. A portion of the orders used at our institution is presented in **Figs. 5** and **6**. For patients undergoing PCI, the ACT can be used to monitor the effect of

---

Box 3
Dosing of DTIs

Argatroban

1. VTE treatment in patients with HIT: 2 μg/kg/min IV infusion

   a. Hepatic impairment: 0.5 μg/kg/min IV infusion

2. For patients with heart failure, multiple organ system failure, severe anasarca, or after cardiac surgery: 0.5–1.2 μg/kg/h IV infusion

Bivalirudin

1. ACS with PCI: bolus of 0.75 mg/kg IV bolus followed by 1.75 mg/kg/h IV infusion

   a. If CrCl <30 mL/min: 0.75 mg/kg IV bolus followed by 1 mg/kg/h IV infusion

   b. Dialysis: 0.75 mg/kg IV bolus followed by 0.25 mg/kg/h IV infusion

2. VTE treatment in patients with HIT: 0.15–0.2 mg/kg/h (non–FDA-approved indication)

   a. If CrCl <30 mL/min: 0.08 mg/kg/h IV infusion

   b. Dialysis: 0.02 mg/kg/h IV infusion

Abbreviations: ACS, acute coronary syndrome; HIT, heparin-induced thrombocytopenia; PCI, percutaneous coronary intervention; VTE, venous thromboembolism.

---

the DTIs.[12] The DTIs can induce a falsely increased international normalized ratio (INR) value, which may alarm clinicians. Argatroban has a much greater effect on the INR than bivalirudin.[1] According to the manufacturer, "DTIs, including argatroban interfere with global tests of coagulation such as the aPTT, PT, INR, ACT, and thrombin time (TT) in a dose dependent fashion. During monotherapy with DTIs and during concurrent therapy with warfarin, INR values are confounded and elevated. The magnitude of INR prolongation from DTIs depends upon both the thromboplastin sensitivity (ISI) as well as the DTI serum concentration. In a retrospective analysis of an argatroban clinical trial, elevated INR values that occurred during therapy with argatroban alone or in combination with warfarin did not result in an increased risk of major bleeding or a difference in efficacy outcomes in patients with HIT." In conclusion, the author would suggest that the INR not be used to manage therapy with argatroban and increases in INR should be disregarded.

Argatroban initial dosing:

☐ **Normal Dosage:**
Argatroban (250 mg in 250 mL 0.9% NaCl = 1 mg/mL) **2 mcg/kg/minute** IV continuous infusion.

☐ **Reduced Dosage:**
Argatroban (250 mg in 250 mL 0.9% NaCl = 1 mg/mL) **0.5 mcg/kg/minute** IV continuous infusion.
- *(i.e., Child-Pugh score greater than 6 or bilirubin greater than 1.5 mg/dL or heart failure or multiple organ system failure or severe anasarca or status-post heart surgery)*

Adjust infusion rate based on table below.

Argatroban Dosing Scale (Target aPTT = 1.5 to 3 x control)		
aPTT Obtained	Infusion Hold Time	Infusion Rate Change
Less than 45 seconds	----	Multiply current rate (mL/hour) by 1.2 for new rate; obtain aPTT in 2 hours
45 - 90 seconds	----	**Continue infusion at the same rate**
Greater than 90 seconds	1 hour	Multiply current rate (mL/hour) by 0.5 for new rate; obtain aPTT 2 hours
MAX DOSE 10 mcg/kg/minute		

Fig. 5. Argatroban weight-based dosing for HIT. (*Courtesy of* The University of Texas MD Anderson Cancer Center, Houston, TX. © 2010; with permission.)

Bivalirudin initial dosing:

☐ <u>**Normal Renal Function (Creatinine Clearance greater than 30 mL/minute):**</u>
  Bivalirudin (250 mg in 250 mL 0.9% NaCl = 1 mg/mL) **0.15 mg/kg/hour** IV continuous infusion
☐ <u>**Moderate Renal Impairment (Creatinine Clearance less than or equal to 30 mL/minute):**</u>
  Bivalirudin (250 mg in 250 mL 0.9% NaCl = 1 mg/mL) **0.08 mg/kg/hour** IV continuous infusion
☐ <u>**Severe Renal Impairment (Dialysis):**</u>
  Bivalirudin (250 mg in 250 mL 0.9% NaCl = 1 mg/mL) **0.02 mg/kg/hour** IV continuous infusion

Adjust infusion rate based on table below.

Bivalirudin Dosing Scale (Target aPTT = 1.5 to 2.5 x control)		
aPTT Obtained	Infusion Hold Time	Infusion Rate Change
Less than 45 seconds	----	Multiply current rate (mL/hour) by 1.2 for new rate; obtain aPTT in 2 hours
45 - 75 seconds	----	**Continue infusion at the same rate**
Greater than 75 seconds	1 hour	Multiply current rate (mL/hour) by 0.5 for new rate; obtain aPTT in 2 hours

Fig. 6. Bivalirudin weight-based dosing for HIT. (*Courtesy of* The University of Texas MD Anderson Cancer Center, Houston, TX. © 2010; with permission.)

Transitioning from argatroban to warfarin once the platelet count has recovered can be difficult because of the falsely increased INR value. The following steps are recommended:

- If the argatroban rate is less than 2 μg/kg/min and the INR is greater than 4. then stop infusion and repeat the INR in 4 hours; if the INR is between 2 and 3, then continue with warfarin monotherapy.
- If the argatroban rate is 2 μg/kg/min or higher, then reduce the rate to 2 μg/kg/min for 4 hours and measure the INR.
  - If the INR is less than 4, continue both and repeat the INR daily until it is greater than 4.
  - If the INR is greater than 4, then stop the argatroban infusion and check the INR in 4 hours:
    - If the INR is between 2 and 3, then continue with warfarin monotherapy.
    - If the INR is less than 2, then restart argatroban and repeat these steps the following day until the INR is between 2 and 3.[13]

Adverse Effects

Bleeding is the most common adverse effect of the DTIs.

Reversal

No antidote is available for reversal of the DTIs; however, their short half-life makes DTIs a favorable option for patients who may be at a high risk of bleeding. If a hemorrhagic event occurs, supportive care treatment such as local hemostasis and blood product administration is recommended. Deamino-D-arginine vasopressin (DDAVP) at doses of 0.3 μg/kg IV over 15 minutes has been shown in experimental models to shorten the bleeding time and reduce the aPTT.[14] Antifibrinolytics such as aminocaproic acid or tranexamic acid may also be considered for life-threatening bleeds.[14]

SUMMARY

Anticoagulation is common in the ICU, but with the use of nurse-driven protocols and safety protocols such as double-checking doses and automated IV pumps, unnecessary adverse events can be avoided. Heparin, LMWHs, and DTIs have advantages and disadvantages for use in critically ill patients. Proper monitoring and knowledge of reversal strategies enhance the likelihood of optimal patient outcomes.

REFERENCES

1. Garcia DA, Baglin TP, Weitz JI, et al. Parenteral anticoagulants: antithrombotic therapy and prevention of thrombosis, 9th ed: American College of Chest Physicians evidence-based clinical practice guidelines. Chest 2012;141(Suppl 2): e24S–43S.
2. Bussey H, Francis JL. Heparin overview and issues. Pharmacotherapy 2004;24(8 Pt 2):103S–7S.
3. Jauch EC, Saver JL, Adams HP Jr, et al. Guidelines for the early management of patients with acute ischemic stroke: a guideline for healthcare professionals from the American Heart Association/American Stroke Association. Stroke 2013;44(3): 870–947.
4. Raschke RA, Reilly BM, Guidry JR, et al. The weight-based heparin dosing nomogram compared with a "standard care" nomogram: a randomized controlled trial. Ann Intern Med 1993;119:874–81.
5. Bernardi E, Piccioli A, Oliboni G, et al. Nomograms for the administration of unfractionated heparin in the initial treatment of acute thromboembolism–an overview. Thromb Haemost 2000;84(1):22–6.
6. Linkins LA, Dans AL, Moores LK, et al. Treatment and prevention of heparin-induced thrombocytopenia: antithrombotic therapy and prevention of thrombosis, 9th ed: American College of Chest Physicians Evidence-Based Clinical Practice Guidelines. Chest 2012;141(Suppl 2):e495S–530S.
7. Hirsh J, Dalen JE, Deykin D, et al. Heparin: mechanism of action, pharmacokinetics, dosing considerations, monitoring, efficacy, and safety. Chest 1992; 102(Suppl 4):337S–51S.
8. Schulman S, Bijsterveld NR. Anticoagulants and their reversal. Transfus Med Rev 2007;21(1):37–48.
9. Levi M, Eerenberg E, Kamphuisen PW. Bleeding risk and reversal strategies for old and new anticoagulants and antiplatelet agents. J Thromb Haemost 2011; 9(9):1705–12.
10. Middeldorp S. Heparin: from animal organ extract to designer drug. Thromb Res 2008;122(6):753–62.
11. Nutescu EA, Spinler SA, Wittkowsky A, et al. Low-molecular-weight heparins in renal impairment and obesity: available evidence and clinical practice recommendations across medical and surgical settings. Ann Pharmacother 2009; 43(6):1064–83.
12. Nutescu EA, Wittkowsky AK. Direct thrombin inhibitors for anticoagulation. Ann Pharmacother 2004;38(1):99–109.
13. Nutescu EA, Shapiro NL, Chevalier A. New anticoagulant agents: direct thrombin inhibitors. Cardiol Clin 2008;26(2):169–87.
14. Crowther MA, Warkentin TE. Bleeding risk and the management of bleeding complications in patients undergoing anticoagulant therapy: focus on new anticoagulant agents. Blood 2008;111(10):4871–9.

Outpatient Management of Oral Anticoagulation in Atrial Fibrillation

Julia A. Manning, MSN, RN, CCRN, ACNP-BC

KEYWORDS

- Atrial fibrillation • Oral anticoagulant • Stroke risk • Treatment • Outpatients

KEY POINTS

- There are currently no head-to-head trials comparing dabigatran, rivaroxaban, and apixaban, and learning to integrate them into clinical practice safely will require time and experience.
- Early follow-up with regular, routine monitoring of compliance, side effects, and renal indices are prudent and are in patients' best interest.
- The results of clinical trials with newer agents have been promising.
- The convenience of newer agents is truly appealing, but their full impact on the reduction of stroke risk and systemic embolism in the setting of atrial fibrillation has yet to be fully realized.

Atrial fibrillation is a commonly encountered problem in the outpatient setting, and brings with it numerous challenges including restoration of a sinus mechanism and the prevention of thromboembolism and stroke.[1] Until recently, the best option for stroke prevention was the initiation of warfarin, a vitamin K antagonist. This approach presented challenges to patients and caregivers alike in the form of numerous food and drug interactions and the need for regular therapeutic monitoring with frequent dose adjustment.[1] Recently, the emergence of target-specific anticoagulants that inhibit either factor Xa or thrombin has given providers safe and effective alternatives to warfarin in the management of patients with new-onset or recurring atrial fibrillation.[2] Providers in the setting of primary care, internal medicine, and cardiology should be well versed in the indications, pharmacokinetics, and side effects of these newer agents, as they can provide patients with better safety, efficacy, and convenience over traditional therapy with warfarin.[3] Formulating the best plan of care for patients with this very common arrhythmia should take into consideration the advantages and disadvantages of each drug, with the ultimate goal being prevention of atrial fibrillation–related stroke.

Woodlands North Houston Heart Center, 411 Lantern Bend Drive, Suite 100, Houston, TX 77090, USA
E-mail address: julie.manning@sbcglobal.net

Crit Care Nurs Clin N Am 25 (2013) 481–487
http://dx.doi.org/10.1016/j.ccell.2013.09.002
0899-5885/13/$ – see front matter © 2013 Elsevier Inc. All rights reserved.

DECIDING TO ANTICOAGULATE

Atrial fibrillation is predicted to affect more than 12 million Americans by the year 2050.[4] The primary concern in these patients is the occurrence of ischemic stroke, which occurs in 15% of patients with atrial fibrillation.[4] There is a 5-fold increased risk of stroke in patients who have had atrial fibrillation. If a patient has had a previous stroke or transient ischemic attack (TIA), their risk of a thromboembolic event is even higher.[4] To help determine stroke-risk stratification many clinicians use the CHADS2 score, a prediction tool that has been previously validated in many clinical trials (**Table 1**).[5] The following risk factors are used: congestive heart failure, hypertension, age 75 years or older, diabetes mellitus, and stroke or TIA. Each of the risk factors counts as 1 point except stroke and TIA, each of which counts as 2 points. A score of 4 or greater is considered high risk, 2 to 3 is considered moderate risk, and less than 2 is considered low risk. In general, anticoagulation with an agent other than aspirin is recommended for patients with a score of 2 or greater.[5] Patients who are at low risk may simply be treated with 81 to 325 mg of aspirin daily.[5]

Previously, warfarin was the mainstay of stroke-prevention therapy in the management of atrial fibrillation. The pharmacokinetics of warfarin is influenced by several factors such as diet, medications, herbal remedies, and genetics.[6] The need for frequent monitoring, coupled with a very narrow therapeutic range and risk of bleeding, makes warfarin a less than desirable choice when deciding on a treatment plan for patients with atrial fibrillation.[5] A therapeutic International Normalized Ratio (INR) cannot be achieved by as many as half of patients taking warfarin despite frequent monitoring.[7] Clinical trial settings have shown patients to be overtreated or undertreated in approximately 4 of 12 months.[8] For elderly patients, frequent monitoring of the INR alone can be a significant deterrent to compliance with prescribed therapy, given the mobility and transportation issues that many face. Home INR monitoring is an option for many patients but requires strict compliance with testing and reporting of results, and can also be cost prohibitive, eliminating many patients as candidates.

The emergence of several target-specific oral anticoagulants (TSOAs) is revolutionizing the way atrial fibrillation is treated in the outpatient setting. TSOAs have given providers and patients better options for stroke prevention, in some cases resulting in an improvement patients' quality of life. In patients with atrial fibrillation, dabigatran, rivaroxaban, and apixaban specifically have been shown to be more efficacious than warfarin in the prevention of stroke and systemic embolism.[9] Monitoring of these agents is not necessary except in patients with renal or hepatic impairment, patients older than 75 years, the very obese, or those with very low body weight.[8] In addition,

Table 1
Calculation of the CHADS2 score[5]

Condition	Points
Congestive heart failure	1
Hypertension (treated with at least 1 medication or blood pressure consistently >140/90 mm Hg)	1
Age >75 y	1
Diabetes mellitus	1
Prior Stroke or transient ischemic attack	2

Score: 4 = high risk; 2–3 = moderate risk; 2 or less = low risk.

TSOAs appear to have a very favorable safety profile and require little or no ongoing monitoring, which makes them an attractive alternative to warfarin.[9]

DABIGATRAN

Dabigatran is an oral, direct thrombin inhibitor, which prevents the conversion of fibrinogen to fibrin and thrombin-inducing platelet aggregation.[3] It is indicated for the treatment of nonvalvular atrial fibrillation. In the noninferiority study Randomized Evaluation of Long-Term Anticoagulation Therapy (RE-LY), dabigatran was compared at 2 fixed doses with dose-adjusted warfarin (INR range 2–3). The study was a randomized, multicenter, open-label trial. Patients with atrial fibrillation and an increased risk of stroke were assigned to one of the treatment groups. Exclusion criteria included patients with a stroke in the last 14 days, a severe stroke in the previous 6 months, major heart-valve disease, any risk factor for hemorrhage, pregnancy, active hepatic disorder, and creatinine clearance (CrCl) of 30 mL/min.[4] Approximately one-third of the patients enrolled had a CHADS2 score of 3 or more. Patients in the warfarin arm were able to achieve therapeutic INR only 64% of the time. In patients randomized to dabigatran 110 mg, the incidence of stroke or systemic embolism was 1.5% per year. For patients randomized to dabigatran 150 mg, the incidence was 1.1% per year compared with 1.7% per year for those in the warfarin group. Occurrence of hemorrhagic stroke was lower with dabigatran (0.12%/y with 110 mg and 0.10%/y with 150 mg vs 0.38%/y with warfarin; $P<.001$) Major bleeding events were similar in the group randomized to dabigatran 150 mg and warfarin (3.11%/y vs 3.36%/y). However, in those patients taking the lower dose of dabigatran, there was a lower incidence of major bleeding events (2.71%) in comparison with patients randomized to warfarin.[10]

Dabigatran is dosed twice daily at 150 mg. Because it is eliminated through the kidneys, patients with renal impairment require dose adjustment based on their CrCl value. No dosage adjustment is necessary for moderate renal impairment (CrCl 30–50 mL/min).[11] For patients with CrCl of 15–30 mL/min, the dose decreases to 75 mg twice daily. Patients with a CrCl of less than 15 mL/min are not candidates for dabigatran.

Several drugs and herbal preparations, such as St John's wort, rifampicin, phenytoin, and phenobarbital, can decrease the plasma concentration of dabigatran. When administered together with dronedarone (Multaq) for the treatment of atrial fibrillation, the concentration of dabigatran is almost 2 times higher. Consequently, the coadministration of these 2 drugs is not recommended.[12]

At present, there is no specific reversal agent for TSOAs. For mild to moderate bleeding, simply stopping the agent is recommended. For severe bleeding, fresh frozen plasma or prothrombin complex concentrates may be of benefit.[11] Hemodialysis can be used for the removal of dabigatran from the blood and, in the case of drug overdosing, activated charcoal may be administered within 3 hours of ingestion of oral anticoagulant intake, which will reduce gastrointestinal absorption.[11]

RIVAROXABAN

Rivaroxaban is an oral factor Xa inhibitor that is indicated for stroke reduction in non-valvular atrial fibrillation,[12] and the treatment of deep venous thrombosis and pulmonary embolism.[11] The pharmacokinetics is stable and dose-dependent, and demonstrates a very quick onset of action of 30 minutes.[11] Its antithrombin effect is secondary to a decrease in the generation of thrombin (through factor Xa inhibition), which results in diminished thrombin-mediated activation of platelets and coagulation.[3] The clinical trial Rivaroxaban Once Daily Oral Direct Factor Xa Inhibition Compared With Vitamin K Antagonism for Prevention of Stroke and Embolism Trial in Atrial Fibrillation (ROCKET-AF) assigned more than 14,000 patients to either rivaroxaban 20 mg daily or dose-adjusted warfarin with a target INR of 2 to 3.[4] This trial was a multicenter randomized study. Patients who had had a previous stroke, TIA, or systemic embolism were included, as were those with at least 2 of the following risk factors: heart failure, left ventricular ejection fraction lower than 35%, hypertension, 75 years of age or older, or diabetes mellitus. Approximately 87% of the patients enrolled had a moderate to high risk of stroke with a mean CHADS2 score of 3.5.[4] Rivaroxaban was found to be noninferior to warfarin for the reduction of stroke and systemic embolism. In the rivaroxaban group, stroke and systemic embolism occurred at a rate of 2.1% per year compared with 2.4% per year in the warfarin group. Major bleeding events and other clinically relevant bleeding was comparable between the 2 groups (14.9%/y in the rivaroxaban group and 14.5%/y year in the warfarin group; $P = .44$). In the rivaroxaban group there were significant reductions in intracranial hemorrhage (0.5% vs 0.7%, $P = .02$) and fatal bleeding (0.2% vs 0.5%, $P = .003$).[13]

As with dabigatran, rivaroxaban is not recommended in patients with a CrCl of less than 15 mL/min. In addition, patients taking azole-antimycotic and human immunodeficiency virus protease inhibitors are not good candidates for rivaroxaban. Rivaroxaban is metabolized in the liver via CYP3A4, which these drugs strongly inhibit.[12] There is currently no antidote or reversal agent for rivaroxaban. In cases of overdose, activated charcoal should be administered; however, hemodialysis has been found to be ineffective, owing to the highly protein-bound characteristic of rivaroxaban. Because it is a factor Xa inhibitor, administering fresh frozen plasma and other similar compounds may help reverse its effects.[12]

APIXABAN

Apixaban is a direct factor Xa inhibitor. Similar to rivaroxaban, it does not require antithrombin for antithrombotic activity and inhibits factor Xa activity that is both free and clot bound.[3] Its only indication is for the prevention of stroke in nonvalvular atrial fibrillation.

The Apixaban for Reduction in Stroke and Other Thrombotic Events In Atrial Fibrillation (ARISTOTLE) trial compared apixaban 5 mg twice daily with dose-adjusted warfarin (target INR 2.0–3.0). More than 18,000 patients were enrolled in this randomized, double-blind, multicenter, noninferiority study.[4] Patients enrolled had documented atrial fibrillation as well as the occurrence of 1 of the following in the previous 12 months: TIA, stroke or thromboembolic event, left ventricular ejection fraction less than 40%, diabetes mellitus, age older than 75 years, or hypertension. Exacerbation of heart failure in the previous 3 months was also an inclusion criterion. Exclusion criteria were stroke in the previous 7 days, major stroke in the previous 6 months, major heart valve disease, CrCl of less than 25 mL/min, currently taking aspirin dose of greater than 165 mg daily, or dual therapy with aspirin and clopidogrel. The mean CHADS2 score for these patients was 2.1. The warfarin group achieved a therapeutic INR range 62% of the time, as was similarly seen in the ROCKET-AF trial of rivaroxaban. The primary outcome was ischemic or hemorrhagic stroke or systemic embolism.

The ARISTOTLE study reported that apixaban was superior to warfarin in preventing stroke in patients with atrial fibrillation. The incidence of the primary outcome was 1.27% in the apixaban group and 1.60% in the warfarin group. Major bleeding occurred at a lower rate in the apixaban group (2.13%/y vs 3.09%/y in the warfarin group). It also outperformed warfarin in decreasing the incidence of intracranial hemorrhage (0.24%/y in the apixaban group and 0.47%/y in the warfarin group; P<.001).[14]

The recommended dose of apixaban for stroke prevention in atrial fibrillation is 5 mg twice daily. Dose reduction to 2.5 mg twice daily is recommended for patients with 2 or more of the following: age 80 years and older, body weight less than 60 kg, or a serum creatinine level greater than 1.5 mg/dL. At present no specific reversal agent for apixaban is available. As is the case for rivaroxaban and dabigatran, in instances of overdosing, activated charcoal should be given.[12]

WHICH DRUG TO CHOOSE?

Preventing stroke in the setting of atrial fibrillation is the primary indication for anticoagulant therapy.[15] With the advent of TSOAs have come more options for providers, and the opportunity to offer their patients optimal stroke protection as well as little interference with quality of life. Three large phase III trials, ROCKET-AF, RE-LY, and ARISTOTLE, have all shown their agents to be noninferior to warfarin for stroke prevention and have also demonstrated fewer intracranial bleeds.[15] These newer agents have also eliminated the need for frequent laboratory testing, which is an attractive option especially for those patients with transportation or mobility issues. However, providers need to consider several points when deciding which oral anticoagulant to prescribe for their patients.

Older patients may experience an increasing effect of the TSOAs in comparison with warfarin, with the exception of dabigatran, which outperformed warfarin in any age group. When evaluating the risk of major bleeding, dabigatran showed the greatest benefit to younger patients. However, both factor Xa inhibitors (rivaroxaban and apixaban) demonstrated reduced stroke risk for older patients in comparison with warfarin.[15] Renal function deficiencies are commonly seen in older patients. None of the newer agents are approved for use in the setting of a CrCl of less than 15 mL/min. However, all three agents may be given at a decreased dose when the Cr/Cl is between 15–30 mL/min. Of the three, Dabigatran is the most dependent on renal function for its elimination.[15]

With newer options available, providers must decide whether to transition patients currently on warfarin therapy to a TSOA. Patients who are likely to benefit from a switch to one of the TSOAs are those who have difficulty getting their INRs to stabilize. Often patients have inconsistent dietary habits or are on chronic medications that easily influence INR levels (ie, antibiotics, acetaminophen). Patients with difficulty traveling for laboratory monitoring may benefit from a medication that does not necessitate frequent testing. However, regardless of the agent compliance is essential, and follow-up, whether in the office or on the phone, may help prevent this issue. For many, the higher cost of these newer agents inhibits the initiation of therapy with 1 of the 3. Older patients are likely already on several other medications that pose a financial burden for them. Choosing a medication that is either not covered on their prescription plan or covered in a higher tier is often not an option. Therefore, the likely choice would be to provide stroke risk reduction with warfarin which is available in generic form and at a much lower cost.[15]

Undoubtedly the major disadvantage of the new oral anticoagulants is the lack of an antidote or reversal agent.[16] Although rivaroxaban and apixaban may be safely discontinued 1 day before elective surgery, urgent surgery poses more of a challenge. Should the need arise, their antithrombotic effect can be reduced in the administration of prothrombin complex concentrates, but this has not definitively been proved to reverse the factor Xa inhibitors.[17] Dabigatran should be stopped 2 days before elective surgery, and in the setting of a CrCl of less than 50 mL/min should be stopped 3 to 5 days before surgery.[4]

Perhaps the most encouraging benefit that has emerged from each of the clinical trials comparing new oral anticoagulants with warfarin is the marked reduction in intracranial hemorrhage in all 3 agents.[16] In RE-LY, ROCKET AF, and ARISTOTLE, the rate of intracranial hemorrhage in the TSOAs versus warfarin was 0.23 versus 0.74 (P<.0001), 0.49 versus 0.74 (P = .019), and 0.33 versus 0.80 (P<.0001), respectively.[16] A commonly encountered fear of patients having to take anticoagulants in any form is the fear of intracranial bleeding. Providers often share their hesitation, but need to provide stroke protection in the most effective manner possible while minimizing their risk for adverse events. Use of one of the new agents offers some reassurance on this front and, it is hoped, will reveal even more benefit as future clinical trials are completed and experience with these agents grows.

In the outpatient setting, it is essential for providers to understand some of the basic indications and dosage considerations when prescribing dabigatran, rivaroxaban, or apixaban for patients with non-valvular atrial fibrillation (**Table 2**). Current evidence suggests that all are at least as effective as, and in some cases superior to warfarin, are practical in their administration, require minimal or no laboratory monitoring, and have very few safety issues.[16] The Canadian Cardiovascular Society update of atrial fibrillation guidelines clearly states that the new TSOAs are preferred to warfarin therapy for the prevention of stroke in patients with atrial fibrillation unless they have maintained a well-controlled INR time in therapeutic range or have a CrCl of less than 30 mL/min.[18] However, despite all of their obvious conveniences and advantages, they are anticoagulants and carry with them an inherent risk of bleeding. Reversibility remains an ongoing issue for these particular agents.

As there are currently no head-to-head trials comparing dabigatran, rivaroxaban, and apixaban, learning to integrate them into clinical practice safely will require time and experience. Early follow-up with regular, routine monitoring of compliance, side effects, and renal indices are prudent and in patients' best interests. The results of clinical trials with these newer agents thus far are promising. Their convenience is truly appealing, but their full impact on the reduction of stroke risk and systemic embolism in the setting of atrial fibrillation has yet to be fully realized.[1]

Table 2 Comparison of Target Specific Oral Anticoagulants			
TSOAs	**Dabigatran**	**Rivaroxaban**	**Apixaban**
Indication	Stroke reduction in nonvalvular atrial fibrillation	Stroke reduction in nonvalvular atrial fibrillation, treatment of DVT and PE	Stroke reduction in nonvalvular atrial fibrillation
Dosage	150 mg BID	20 mg QD	5 mg BID
Target	Direct thrombin inhibitor	Factor Xa inhibitor	Factor Xa inhibitor
Renal dosing	75 mg BID Avoid use in CrCl <15 mL/min	15 mg QD Avoid use in CrCl <15 mL/min	2.5 mg BID Avoid use in CrCl <15 mL/min
Converting from warfarin	Wait to start until INR <2.0	Wait to start until INR <3.0	Wait to start until INR <2.0

Abbreviations: BID, twice daily; CrCl, creatinine clearance; DVT, deep venous thrombosis; INR, International Normalized Ratio; PE, pulmonary embolus; QD, once daily.

REFERENCES

1. Mantha S, Cabral K, Ansell J. New avenues for anticoagulation in atrial fibrillation. Clin Pharmacol Ther 2013;93:68–77.
2. Konkle B. Monitoring target specific anticoagulants. J Thromb Thrombolysis 2013;35:387–90.
3. Norgard N, DiNicolantonio J, Topping T, et al. Novel anticoagulants in atrial fibrillation stroke prevention. Ther Adv Chronic Dis 2013;3:123–36.
4. O'Dell K, Igawa D, Hsin J. New oral anticoagulants for atrial fibrillation: a review of clinical trials. Clin Ther 2012;34:894–901.
5. Gutierrez C, Blanchard D. Atrial fibrillation: diagnosis and treatment. Am Fam Physician 2011;83:61–8.
6. Dittus C, Ansell J. The evolution of oral anticoagulation therapy. Prim Care 2013; 40:109–34.
7. Baker W, Cios D, Sander S, et al. Meta-analysis to assess the quality of warfarin control in atrial fibrillation patients in the United States. J Manag Care Pharm 2009;15:244–52.
8. Mani H, Kasper A, Lindhoff-Last E. Measuring the anticoagulant effects of target specific oral anticoagulants-reasons, methods and current limitations. J Thromb Thrombolysis 2013;36(2):187–94. Available at: https://www.ncbi.nlm.nih.gov/pubmed/23512159. Accessed April 16, 2013.
9. Miller C, Grandi S, Shimony A, et al. Meta-analysis of efficacy and safety of new oral anticoagulants (dabigatran, rivaroxaban, apixaban) versus warfarin in patients with atrial fibrillation. Am J Cardiol 2012;110(3):453–60. Available at: http://dx.doi.org/10.1016/j.amjcard.2012.03.049. Accessed April 16, 2013.
10. Connolly S, Ezekowitz M, Yusuf S, et al. Dabigatran versus warfarin in patients with atrial fibrillation. N Engl J Med 2009;362:1139–51.
11. Tun N, Oo T. Prevention and treatment of venous thromboembolism with new oral anticoagulants: a practical update for clinicians. Thrombosis 2013;2013:183616. Available at: http://dx.doi.org/10.1155/2013/183616. Accessed April 16, 2013.
12. Caterina R, Husted S, Wallentin L, et al. New oral anticoagulants in atrial fibrillation and acute coronary syndromes. J Am Coll Cardiol 2012;59:1413–25.
13. Patel M, Mahaffey K, Garg J, et al. Rivaroxaban versus warfarin in nonvalvular atrial fibrillation. N Engl J Med 2011;365:883–91.
14. Granger C, Alexander J, McMurray J, et al. Apixaban versus warfarin in patients with atrial fibrillation. N Engl J Med 2011;365:981–92.
15. Schulman S. New anticoagulants in atrial fibrillation management. Thromb Res 2013;131(Suppl 1):S63–6.
16. Becattini C, Vedovati M, Agnelli G. Old and new oral anticoagulants for venous thromboembolism and atrial fibrillation: a review of the literature. Thromb Res 2012;129:392–400.
17. Yeung L, Miraflor E, Harken A. Confronting the chronically anticoagulated, acute care surgery patient as we evolve into the post-warfarin era. Surgery 2012;153: 308–15.
18. Skanes A. Focused 2012 update of the Canadian Cardiovascular Society atrial fibrillation guidelines: recommendations for stroke prevention and rate/rhythm control. Can J Cardiol 2012;28:125–36.

Index

Note: Page numbers of article titles are in **boldface** type.

Crit Care Nurs Clin N Am 25 (2013) 489–494
http://dx.doi.org/10.1016/S0899-5885(13)00097-X
0899-5885/13/$ – see front matter © 2013 Elsevier Inc. All rights reserved.
ccnursing.theclinics.com

United States Postal Service

Statement of Ownership, Management, and Circulation
(All Periodicals Publications Except Requestor Publications)

1. Publication Title	2. Publication Number								3. Filing Date
Critical Care Nursing Clinics of North America	0	0	6	-	2	7	3		9/14/13

4. Issue Frequency	5. Number of Issues Published Annually	6. Annual Subscription Price
Mar, Jun, Sep, Dec	4	$144.00

7. Complete Mailing Address of Known Office of Publication (Not printer) (Street, city, county, state, and ZIP+4®)

Elsevier Inc.
360 Park Avenue South
New York, NY 10010-1710

Contact Person
Stephen R. Bushing
Telephone (Include area code)
215-239-3688

8. Complete Mailing Address of Headquarters or General Business Office of Publisher (Not printer)

Elsevier Inc., 360 Park Avenue South, New York, NY 10010-1710

9. Full Names and Complete Mailing Addresses of Publisher, Editor, and Managing Editor (Do not leave blank)

Publisher (Name and complete mailing address)

Linda Belfus, Elsevier, Inc., 1600 John F . Kennedy Blvd. Suite 1800, Philadelphia, PA 19103-2899

Editor (Name and complete mailing address)

Katie Saunders, Elsevier, Inc., 1600 John F. Kennedy Blvd. Suite 1800, Philadelphia, PA 19103-2899

Managing Editor (Name and complete mailing address)

Adrianne Brigido, Elsevier, Inc., 1600 John F. Kennedy Blvd. Suite 1800, Philadelphia, PA 19103-2899

10. Owner (Do not leave blank. If the publication is owned by a corporation, give the name and address of the corporation immediately followed by the names and addresses of all stockholders owning or holding 1 percent or more of the total amount of stock. If not owned by a corporation, give the names and addresses of the individual owners. If owned by a partnership or other unincorporated firm, give its name and address as well as those of each individual owner. If the publication is published by a nonprofit organization, give its name and address.)

Full Name	Complete Mailing Address
Wholly owned subsidiary of	1600 John F. Kennedy Blvd., Ste. 1800
Reed/Elsevier, US holdings	Philadelphia, PA 19103-2899

11. Known Bondholders, Mortgagees, and Other Security Holders Owning or Holding 1 Percent or More of Total Amount of Bonds, Mortgages, or Other Securities. If none, check box ☑ None

Full Name	Complete Mailing Address
N/A	

12. Tax Status (For completion by nonprofit organizations authorized to mail at nonprofit rates) (Check one)
The purpose, function, and nonprofit status of this organization and the exempt status for federal income tax purposes:
☐ Has Not Changed During Preceding 12 Months
☐ Has Changed During Preceding 12 Months (Publisher must submit explanation of change with this statement)

PS Form 3526, September 2007 (Page 1 of 3 (Instructions Page 3)) PSN 7530-01-000-9931 PRIVACY NOTICE: See our Privacy policy in www.usps.com

---

13. Publication Title			14. Issue Date for Circulation Data Below
Critical Care Nursing Clinics of North America			September 2013

15. Extent and Nature of Circulation			Average No. Copies Each Issue During Preceding 12 Months	No. Copies of Single Issue Published Nearest to Filing Date
a. Total Number of Copies (Net press run)			505	528
b. Paid Circulation (By Mail and Outside the Mail)	(1)	Mailed Outside-County Paid Subscriptions Stated on PS Form 3541. (Include paid distribution above nominal rate, advertiser's proof copies, and exchange copies)	342	390
	(2)	Mailed In-County Paid Subscriptions Stated on PS Form 3541 (Include paid distribution above nominal rate, advertiser's proof copies, and exchange copies)		
	(3)	Paid Distribution Outside the Mails Including Sales Through Dealers and Carriers, Street Vendors, Counter Sales, and Other Paid Distribution Outside USPS®	63	66
	(4)	Paid Distribution by Other Classes Mailed Through the USPS (e.g. First-Class Mail®)		
c. Total Paid Distribution (Sum of 15b (1), (2), (3), and (4))			405	456
d. Free or Nominal Rate Distribution (By Mail and Outside the Mail)	(1)	Free or Nominal Rate Outside-County Copies Included on PS Form 3541	41	37
	(2)	Free or Nominal Rate In-County Copies Included on PS Form 3541		
	(3)	Free or Nominal Rate Copies Mailed at Other Classes Through the USPS (e.g. First-Class Mail)		
	(4)	Free or Nominal Rate Distribution Outside the Mail (Carriers or other means)		
e. Total Free or Nominal Rate Distribution (Sum of 15d (1), (2), (3) and (4))			41	37
f. Total Distribution (Sum of 15c and 15e)			446	493
g. Copies not Distributed (See instructions to publishers #4 (page #3))			59	35
h. Total (Sum of 15f and g)			505	528
i. Percent Paid (15c divided by 15f times 100)			90.81%	92.49%

16. Publication of Statement of Ownership
☐ If the publication is a general publication, publication of this statement is required. Will be printed ☐ Publication not required
in the December 2013 issue of this publication.

17. Signature and Title of Editor, Publisher, Business Manager, or Owner

[signature] Stephen R. Bushing – Inventory Distribution Coordinator
Date September 14, 2013

I certify that all information furnished on this form is true and complete. I understand that anyone who furnishes false or misleading information on this form or who omits material or information requested on the form may be subject to criminal sanctions (including fines and imprisonment) and/or civil sanctions (including civil penalties).

PS Form 3526, September 2007 (Page 2 of 3)

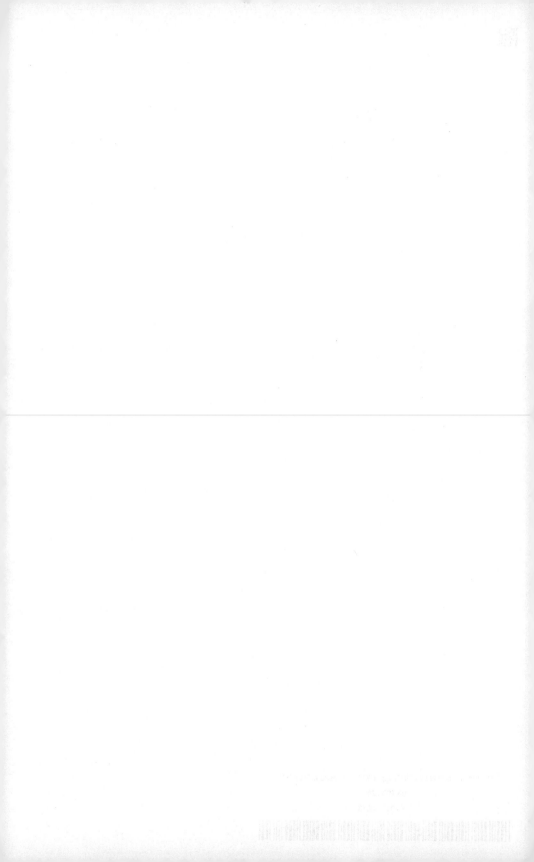

Printed and bound by CPI Group (UK) Ltd, Croydon, CR0 4YY

03/10/2024

01040490-0013